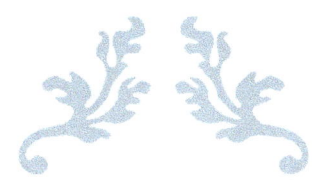

MEDITERRANEAN REFRESH RECIPES

SIMPLE AND EASY MEDITERRANEAN COOKBOOK FOR EVERYONE

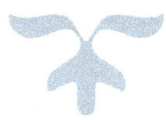

SANDRA RAMOS

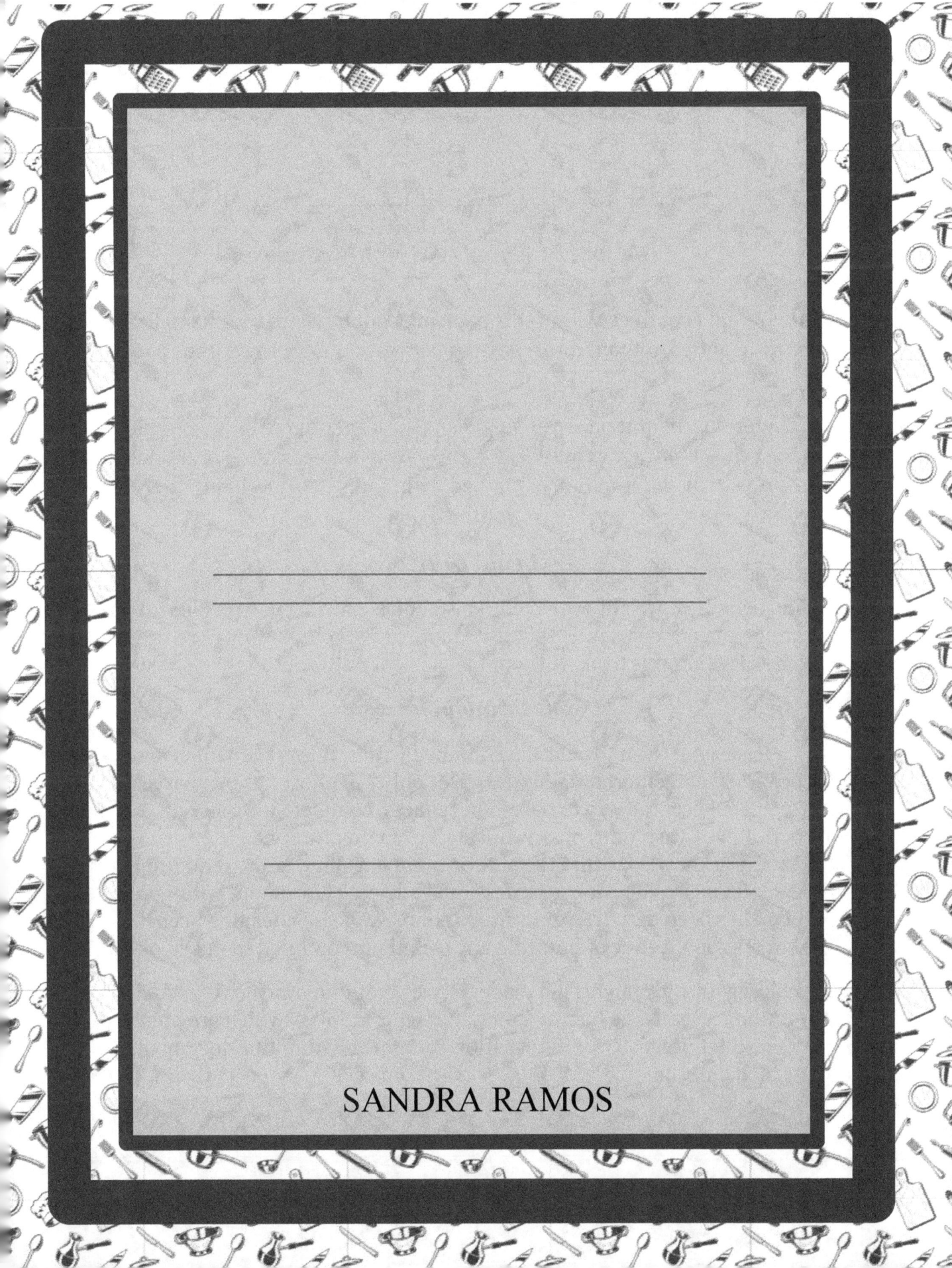

SANDRA RAMOS

Copyright - 2021 - All rights reserved.

The content contained within this book may not be reproduced, duplicated or transmitted without direct written permission from the author or the publisher.

Under no circumstances will any blame or legal responsibility be held against the publisher, or author, for any damages, reparation, or monetary loss due to the information contained within this book, either directly or indirectly.

Legal Notice:

This book is copyright protected. This book is only for personal use. You cannot amend, distribute, sell, use, quote or paraphrase any part, or the content within this book, without the consent of the author or publisher.

Disclaimer Notice:

Please note the information contained within this document is for educational and entertainment purposes only. All effort has been executed to present accurate, up to date, and reliable, complete information. No warranties of any kind are declared or implied.
Readers acknowledge that the author is not engaging in the rendering of legal, financial, medical or professional advice. The content within this book has been derived from various sources. Please consult a licensed professional before attempting any techniques outlined in this book.

By reading this document, the reader agrees that under no circumstances is the author responsible for any losses, direct or indirect, which are incurred as a result of the use of information contained within this document, including, but not limited to, - errors, omissions, or inaccuracies.

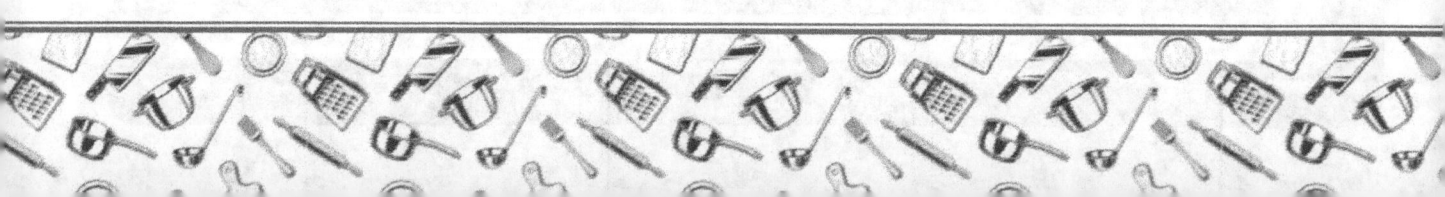

Table of Contents

INTRODUCTION 1

Chapter 1: Why this type of diet is the right for you? 5

Chapter 2: Your Mindset and this diet 9

Chapter 4: Exercise 15

Chapter 5: The recipes in this book 16

Fruits and Desserts 18

    Apricot Spoon Sweets 18

    Pecan Bread with Cherries 19

    Filled Apricots with Rose Water and Pistachios 20

    Peaches and Cherries Poached in Spiced Red Wine 21

    Pears in Oven with Dried Apricots and Pistachios 22

    Apricot Spoon Sweets 23

    Poached Pears with Lemon, Herbs and White Whine 24

    Melon, Plums, and Cherries with Mint and Vanilla 25

    Fruit Mixture with Basil and Pepper 26

    Biscotti with Lemon 27

    Biscotti with Honey and Lavender 28

    Lemon Rice Pudding from Greece 29

    Raspberry Sorbet 30

    Lemon Ice with Mint 31

    Orange Ice with Mint 32

Vanilla Baked Pears 33

Dark Chocolate Fruit Kebabs 34

Butter Cookies 35

Strawberry Tiramisu 36

Spicy Biscotti 37

Honey-Glazed Peaches with Hazelnuts 38

Plums in Oven with Dried Cherries and Almonds 39

Balsamic Strawberries 40

Pignoli 41

Fig Phyllo Cookies 42

Almond Cake 43

Polenta Cake 44

Olive Oil–Yogurt Cake 45

Lemon Mousse with Blueberry Sauce 46

Baklava 47

Lemon Yogurt Mousse with Strawberry Sauce 48

Almonds and Dates Semolina Pudding 49

Lemon Ice 50

Cake for New Year's 51

Banana Sour Cream Bread 52

Pears Filled with Almonds 53

Smoothies 54

Mango Pear Smoothie 54

Lemon and Strawberries Smoothie 55

Orange-Pineapple Smoothie 56

Pineapple Orange Smoothie	57
Peach Smoothie	58
Pear and Strawberries Smoothie	59
Strawberry R. Smoothie	60
Peanut Butter Smoothie	61
Nectarine Smoothie	62
Pineapple Ginger Smoothie	63
Orange and Strawberry Smoothie	64
Melon Mint Smoothie	65
Pineapple Berry Smoothie	66
Papaya Smoothie	67
Coconut Smoothie	68
Pistachio Smoothie	69
Oatmeal Smoothie	70
Orange Coconut Smoothie	71
Peach Cinnamon Smoothie	72
Raspberry Peach Smoothie	73
Fruit Smoothie	74
Apple Coconut Smoothie	75
High Fiber Smoothie	76
Apple Smoothie	77
Triple Fruit Smoothie	78
Strawberry Lemon Smoothie	79
Morning Smoothie	80
Pumpkin Smoothie	81

Paradise Smoothie	82
Honey Lime Fruit Cake	83
Orange Smoothie	84
Banana Pineapple Smoothie	85
Cappuccino Smoothie	86
Peach Apple Smoothie	87
Mousse Mango	88

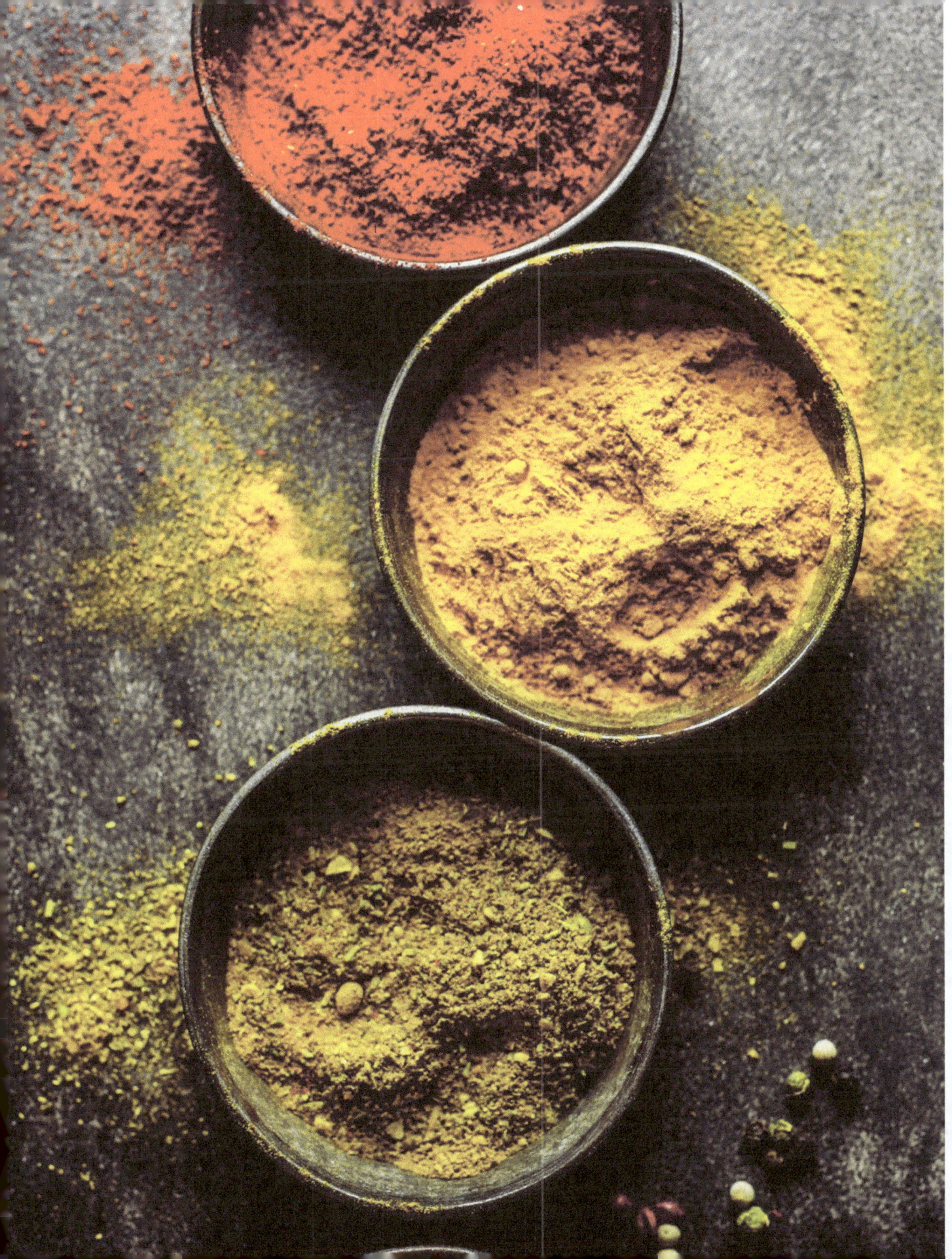

INTRODUCTION

The joy that I am feeling right now cannot be explained. This is because you have chosen me and this book as a guide to a new path – the Mediterranean one. The Mediterranean diet is like no other diet in this world and this way of eating is offering many health and weight benefits.

Right after World War II, Ancel Keys, a scientist and his colleague Paul Dudley, later known as President Eisenhower's cardiac physician made a Seven Countries Study together with couple of their colleagues. They included people from United States and people from Crete – Mediterranean island. The study was testing these people of all ages and Keys implemented the Mediterranean diet in this study as well.

The 13,000 men came from Netherlands, United States, Greece, Italy, Yugoslavia and Japan and it was estimated that fruits, vegetables, grains, beans and fish are the healthiest ingredients ever. This applies even after considering the impoverishment of WWII. Interestingly this was also estimated at the start, imagine what else they discovered.

Among everything else it was discovered that Mediterranean way of food consumption can make one person lose and maintain healthy weight. Every chapter included in this book will reveal different story about this diet plan and how can you become able to change your eating patterns. Also, you will find out that Mediterranean diet plan gives extreme amount of energy and you will become motivated

Chapter 1: Why this type of diet is the right for you?

Simply because it contains healthy plant foods and it is low in animal foods. Unlike other diets, Mediterranean diet offers more seafood and fish. Seafood and fish are way better than any other meat and the benefits of them is visible after a week or two of constant consumption. Plus, Mediterranean recipes do not leave you hungry, you are full after eating for a longer period.

With constant exercise and fruits, vegetables, legumes, nuts and whole grains (everything that this diet is) you will become the best version of yourself without doubt. Also, you will learn how to perfectly switch bad ingredients with good ingredients. For example, instead of butter you will start using canola or olive oil. Instead of salt you will start using different herbs and spices. Print out the Mediterranean pyramid of foods and you won't regret it.

These recipes are family friendly and you'll be able to host and enjoy and host many gatherings with your friends as well because they are also friend friendly. Occasional glass of red wine is okay, so you are good to go.

HEALTH BENEFITS

Healthy fats are the key component when it comes to Mediterranean cuisine. Also, let's not forget about the most important thing this diet has – plant-based food. Yes, this diet does not remove many food groups, but the mixture of ingredients won't make you a single problem and you will learn what goes with what in time.

But let's elaborate on the health benefits a little bit more. It is scientifically proven that the Mediterranean diet is able to lower the risk of strokes and heart disease. Every patient that has used this diet style so far, has shown lowered levels of oxidized low-density lipoprotein or LDL cholesterol (the bad cholesterol which gets build up in your arteries and causes problems with your heart.

NO MORE HEART PROBLEMS AND STROKES

One of the main ingredients in the Mediterranean diet, extra virgin olive oil, contains alpha-linolenic acid and the Warwick Medical School delivered a study that indicated how olive oil is able to decrease blood pressure. Not only that but also the olive oil is able to lower hypertension because it keeps human arteries clearer and more dilated. Also, it makes the nitric oxide more bioavailable and you won't have problems with cholesterol levels anymore. Only if of course, you consume olive oil (extra virgin) on regular bases.

If you are feeling numbness, weakness, headaches, confusion, vision problems, dizziness or slurred speech do not worry no more. This diet helps and improves this condition together with the ultimate problem – strokes that are happening due to bleeding in the brain or blocked blood vessel.

IMPROVED VISION

Another thing that would improve after starting with this diet is your vision. This diet will help you prevent or stave off the risk of macular degeneration which happens to adults over 54. This disease brings blindness and occurs to over 10 million Americans. Imagine the benefit in here, imagine being victorious against something that is able to destroy your retina and remove the chance of clear vision. The vegetables this diet promotes, the green leafy ones have lutein and that lowers the chance of experiencing cataracts as well.

WEIGHT LOSS

You probably want to lose weight as well and the search for the perfect diet that will be able to provide you that is endless. Until now. This diet is also able to give you the chance to lose weight naturally and easily with nutrient rich foods. The focus in here is on healthy fats while carbohydrates are not that present. They are still here as pasta or bread of course, but their implementation is generally low. The healthy fats, protein and fiber will allow you to lose weight and at the same time will keep you satisfied. Thanks to these nutrients you won't have cravings for candy, chips or cookies no more. The vegetables that you'll consume will fill your stomach and you won't feel hunger for hours. You won't even experience spike in your blood sugar.

IMPROVED AGILITY

According to studies, 70 percent of the seniors who have risk of developing frailty or other muscle weakness lowered the factors of experiencing that by implementing this diet in their lives.

YOU'LL START ENJOYING NATURAL FOODS

This is probably the best thing that this diet brings because it is kind of a new characteristic that you'll develop. As previously noted, this diet is low in sugar and processed foods so its recipes will bring you closer to organic produced foods thus closer to nature. For example, this diet offers honey instead of sugar and this change is priceless.

IMPROVED ASTHMA SYMPTOMS

Another study which included children revealed that antioxidant diet is able to help them decrease their asthma symptoms and at the same time made them not like eating a food that is quite popular – red meat. Yes, this diet helps children to say no to red meat and yes to plant-based food.

NO MORE ALZHEIMER'S RISK

Those people that choose this diet plant without doubt lower their risk of getting Alzheimer's disease in the future. In fact, the latest study shows that getting Alzheimer's is reduced by 40 percent to those people that consume Mediterranean diet foods. Additional exercises are recommended in the process as well.

HELPS PEOPLE WITH DIABETES

Excessive insulin is controlled with Mediterranean diet. Not every diet is able to do this and not every diet can control blood sugar levels and control your weight at the same time. As I told before this diet is at the same time low in sugar and high in healthy acids. This makes a balance for your body and burns fat while gives you energy at the same time.

The American Heart Association reveals that this diet unlike other diets is low in saturated fat while high in fat. This keeps your hunger under control and delivers amazing weight loss results.

MEDITERRANEAN DIET HELPS YOUR BRAIN

Sugar is usually responsible for the highs and lows when it comes to your mood. This diet does not contain artificial sugar at all this your mood and overall brain health will improve as well.

THE WEIGHT LOSS JOURNEY

Planning breakfast, lunch or dinner is not hard, but the part gets tricky when it comes to snacking time. You should make something for yourself that contains from 150 to 200 calories. For example, you can choose apple, pear, grapefruit and a pinch of salt.

The path that this diet offers is the safest when it comes to losing weight. Everything is healthy here and there won't be bouncing.

But many people ask what happens when the time is stumbling on us and when we do not have time to cook the meals present in here. Well, I and this diet of course have a solution for you. Trust me you will like it.

- Fruit slices – pears and apples
- Nut butter – cashew butter, almond butter and more
- Dates and figs
- Tuna salad
- Crackers
- Greek Yogurt
- Olives
- Pitas
- Hummus

Chapter 2: Your Mindset and this diet

In order to remove the unwanted pounds, you have to set your mindset on it like never before. Do not think about that all the time, start thinking about something entirely else while you are focused on losing weight. Or in other words, keep yourself busy while you consume Mediterranean diet foods and you regularly exercise. Also do not expect quick fixes. Time is all you need and after successfully sticking to the plant you'll start to realize the change and how big it is.

To be sincere, the Mediterranean diet is the one thing that you have been missing for so long. You are already motivated I think so all you have to do is start. You already purchased this book, so you are on the right path.

Write down your reasons for starting this journey and every time you are feeling down, or you lack motivated read them out loud. Write down your goals as well. Start with something small and increase as time passes.

Another important thing that people usually forget are their surroundings. It is important for you to surround with people that are positive. Positive mindset regardless of what you do is important, especially when it comes to losing weight and changing something as diet pattern. This is how you'll become able to develop emotionally, healthy realistic goals (do not forget to set your goals first).

Focus on your sleep and develop a healthy sleeping pattern as well. Recharging and sleeping for more than 7 hours are essential when it comes to weight loss because you need extreme amount of energy and sharpness. Good energy and brain sharpness appear only when one is able to properly relax and recharge in the evening hours.

Chapter 3: Nutrition and Portions

Start being aware of the things you consume now. Develop your management skills and stick to the guidelines that this book gives. What to consume? Well start with:

- Vegetables – raw and leafy
- Fruit
- Legumes
- Grains (one slice of bread is allowed)
- Dairy
- Meat
- Potatoes
- Nuts

This is the food you must start combining and portions that include these ingredients will make you set and ready for reaching your goals.

This is a sustainable diet so you won't have serious problems, but I will be lying if I say that cravings won't appear. If you successfully understand your cravings, you'll remove them and soon be proud of your dietary success. Remember, cravings for certain foods indicate need of something entirely else, something that your body is need of.

So, the adjustments that you have to make regarding the cravings are:

- Remove salty cravings with couple of nuts or seeds because your body want silicon.

- Remove fatty and oily foods with spinach, broccoli, cheese and fish because your body wants calcium and chloride.

- Remove sugary foods with chicken, beef, lamb, liver, cheese, cauliflower and broccoli because your body wants phosphorous and tryptophan.

- Remove chocolate cravings (this is the hardest one) with spinach, nuts, seeds, broccoli and cheese because your body wants magnesium and chromium.

You also have to:

- Learn how to recognize every healthy ingredient on the labels. Take back everything that does not look good to your or that indicates that there are many artificial preservatives present.

- Check your serving size.

- Always calculate your calories intake

- Consume food rich in calcium, iron, fiber, vitamin A and vitamin C.

Do not consume:

- Added sugar or foods like candy, soda, ice cream and more.

- Refined oils – soybean oil, canola oil cottonseed oil and more.

- Trans fats – margarine, soda, processed meats, beverages, table sugar and more.

- Processed meat.

- Refined grains.

Foods that you should consume:

- Seafood and Fish: Mussels, clams, crab, prawns, oysters, shrimp, tuna, mackerel, salmon, trout, sardines, anchovies, and more

- Poultry: Turkey, duck, chicken, and more

- Eggs: Duck, quail, and chicken eggs

- Dairy Products: Contain calcium, B12, and Vitamin A: Greek yogurt, regular yogurt, cheese, plus others

- Tubers: Yams, turnips, potatoes, sweet potatoes, etc.

- Vegetables: Another excellent choice for fiber, and antioxidants: Cucumbers, carrots, Brussels sprouts, tomatoes, onions, broccoli, cauliflower, spinach, kale, eggplant, artichokes, fennel, etc.

- Seedsand Nuts: Provide minerals, vitamins, fiber, and protein: Macadamia nuts, cashews, pumpkin seeds, sunflower seeds, hazelnuts, chestnuts, Brazil nuts, walnuts, almonds, pumpkin seeds, sesame, poppy, and more

- Fruits: Excellent choices for vitamin C, antioxidants, and fiber: Peaches, bananas, apples, figs, dates, pears, oranges, strawberries, melons, grapes, etc.

- Spices and Herbs: Cinnamon, garlic, pepper, nutmeg, rosemary, sage, mint, basil, parsley, etc.

- Whole Grains: Whole grain bread and pasta, buckwheat, whole wheat, barley, corn, whole oats, rye, quinoa, bulgur, couscous 18

- Legumes: Provide vitamins, fiber, carbohydrates, and protein: Chickpeas, pulses, beans, lentils, peanuts, peas

- Healthy Fats: Avocado oil, avocados, olive oil, olive oil products and olives

- Beverages: Water and tea

- White meat: Consume them but remove the visible fat and skin

- Red meat: You can consume lamb, pork, and beef in small amounts

- Potatoes: Prepare them with caution but consume them because they are excellent source of potassium, vitamin b, vitamin c and fibers.

- Desserts and sweets: consume cakes, biscuits and sweets in extra small amounts.

There is one thing that you can implement that will make your journey even more beautiful – spices and herbs! Traditional Mediterranean diet is filled with different spices and herbs and each has a different health benefit! Believe it or not herbs and spices are able to do that and that is one of the main reasons why people implement them in their diet. Here are the spices you must include and the benefits they bring:

- Anise – improves digestion, reduces nausea and alleviates cramps.
- Bay leaf – treats migraines.
- Basil – aids digestion and reduces anxiety and stress.
- Black pepper – promotes nutrient absorption and speeds up your metabolism.
- Cayenne pepper – increases metabolism and controls your appetite.
- Sweet and spicy cloves – relive pain, gum and tooth pain. Also, kill bacteria, fungal infections and aid digestive problems.
- Fennel – improves bone health.
- Garlic – improves blood sugar levels and helps you lose weight.
- Ginger – serves as diuretic and increases urine elimination.
- Marjoram – promotes healthy digestion and fights type 2 diabetes.
- Mint – treats nasal congestion, nausea, dizziness and headaches.
- Oregano – treats common cold and reduces infections. It also relieves menstrual pain.
- Parsley – improves your skin, prostate, dental health and blood circulation.
- Rosemary – increases hair growth, reduces stress, inflammation and improves pain.
- Sage – improves your digestion problems.
- Thyme – has antibacterial properties.

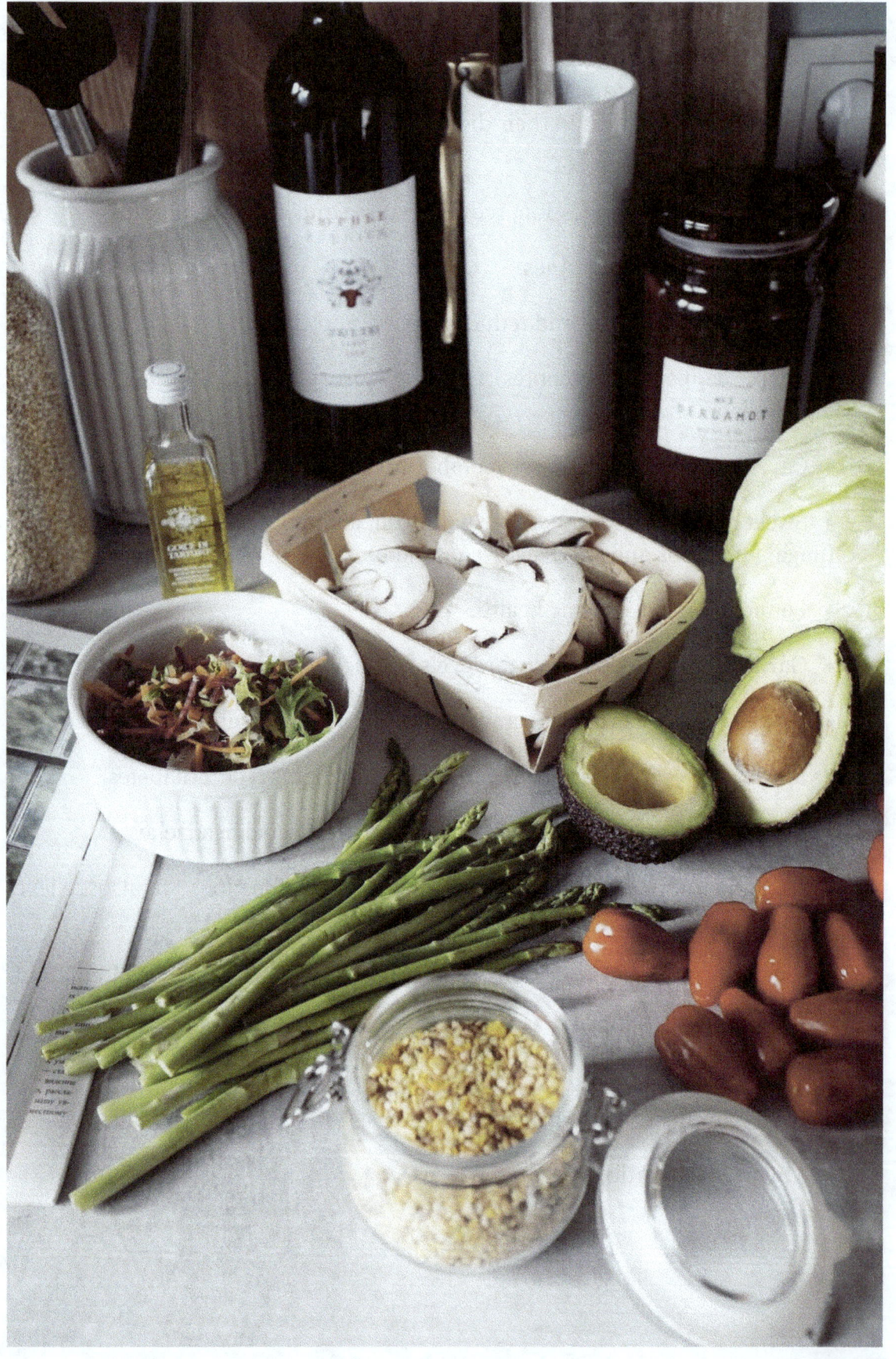

Chapter 4: Exercise

Mediterranean diet is extremely flexible, and you won't have problems while being out with friends. Many recipes in the restaurants come from this particular diet so, you are good to go as long as you do not eat junk food and food that is high in sugar.

Eat slowly and chew your food better. Put your utensils down between bites because that is going to help you slow down the process of eating.

The tips above will help you a lot, but nothing will help you more in this journey than exercising. Two years ago, one scientific research that mainly focused on the Mediterranean diet revealed that this diet is extremely beneficial and gets its full potential when exercise is included. So, to keep your weight under control and to lose weight at the same time you must exercise.

Do not force yourself, start with something easy and small. Spend 30 to 60 minutes daily on that part. Walk, run, do yoga, swim, ride a bike, or simply infiltrate yourself into a regular exercise program online or in a gym near you.

Regular physical activity does not improve only your look, it also improves your strength, mood and balance.

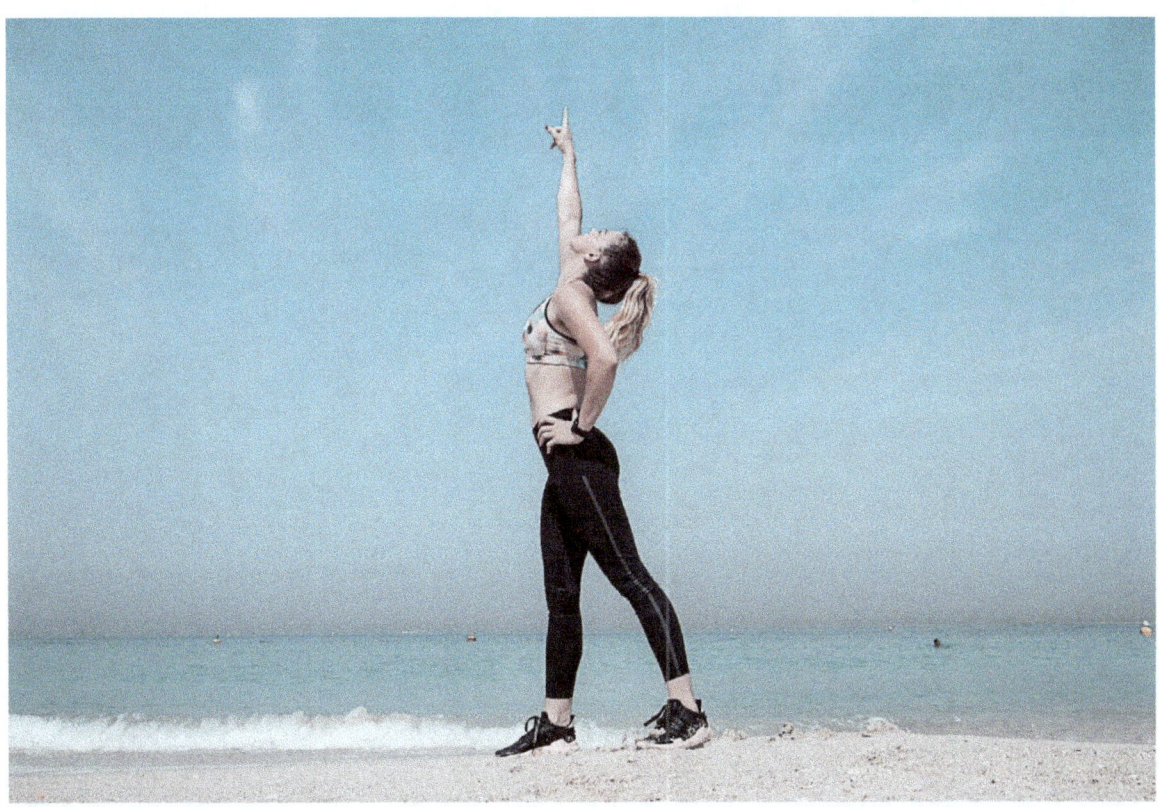

Chapter 5: The recipes in this book

This book contains 500 recipes in total. Each recipe is designed according to the rules Mediterranean diet has. Every recipe is healthy, and every recipe should be made with the best ingredients available – the organic ones. There is also a section for vegans and vegetarians. We wanted to include every person possible in this journey because this journey is all about health and improving yourself and the way you eat. At the bottom of this book you will find a meal plan that we think is going to help you a lot in the few first months. The start won't be that hard, but it is going to be challenging I must admit.

The cooking skills

It is important to know that the Mediterranean do not require hours and hours in the kitchen. The way these recipes are prepared is easy and convenient.

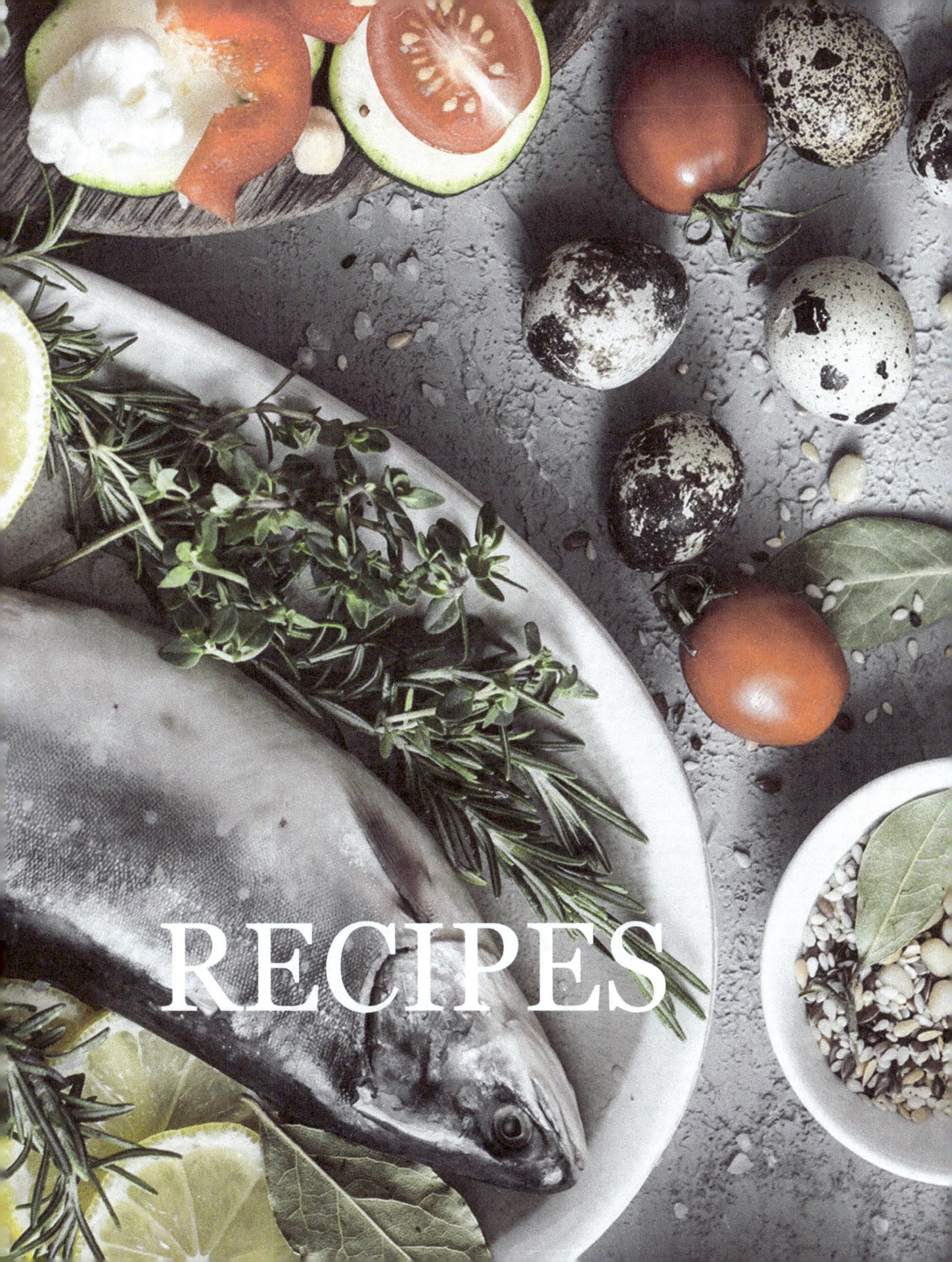

Fruits and Desserts

Apricot Spoon Sweets

COOKING: 40+ MIN

SERVES: 4 Cup

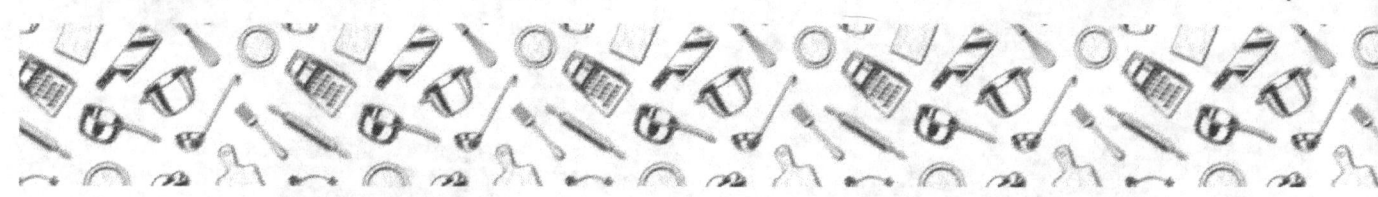

INGREDIENTS

1½ cups sugar
1 cup honey
¾ cup water
1½ pounds ripe but firm apricots, pitted and cut into ½-inch wedges
2 tablespoons lemon juice

Nutritional Value: 313 calories per serving

DIRECTIONS

1. Boil honey, sugar and water over high heat and cook it for 10 minutes with constant stirring.
2. Remove from heat, pour lemon juice and apricots and bring it to boil once again but this time on medium-low heat for 5 minutes.
3. Remove from heat and let it cool.
4. Refrigerate and serve.

Fruits and Desserts

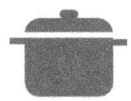

Pecan Bread with Cherries

COOKING: 40+ MIN

SERVES: 4

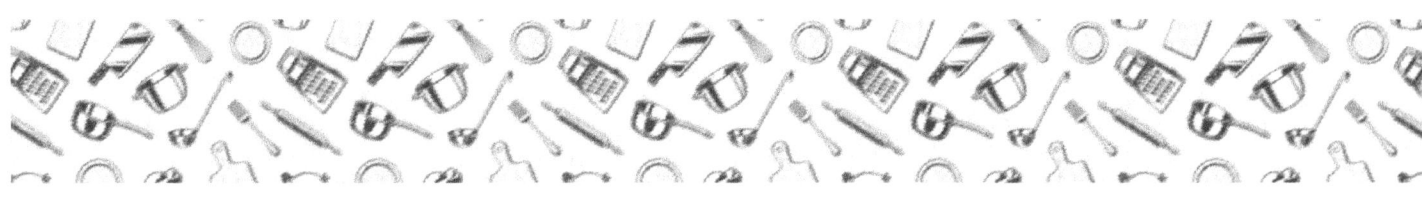

INGREDIENTS

4 cups water
3 tablespoons honey
2 (2-inch) strips lemon zest plus 1 tablespoon juice
2 cinnamon sticks
1¼ teaspoons ground coriander
2 cups (12 ounces) dried figs
¾ cup dried apricots
½ cup dried cherries

Nutritional Value: 369 calories per serving

DIRECTIONS

1. Mix honey, lemon zest, water, lemon juice, coriander and cinnamon sticks and bring it to boil over medium high heat. Cook for 3 to 4 minutes with constant stirring.
2. Add in the apricots and figs. Continue boiling for 30 minutes but this time on medium-low heat.
3. After 30 minutes, add the cherries and cook the mixture until they are plump – approximately 20 minutes. Remove from heat and take out the lemon zest and cinnamon sticks.

Fruits and Desserts

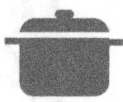 Filled Apricots with Rose Water and Pistachios

COOKING: 40+ MIN   SERVES: 4

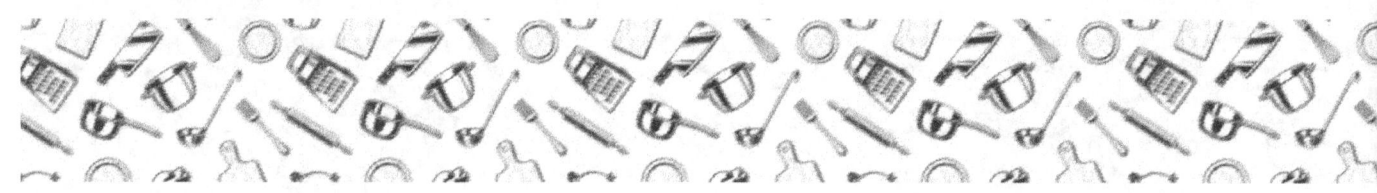

INGREDIENTS

½ cup plain Greek yogurt
¼ cup sugar
½ teaspoon rose water
½ teaspoon grated lemon zest plus 1 tablespoon juice
Salt
2 cups water
4 green cardamom pods, cracked
2 bay leaves
24 whole dried apricots
¼ cup shelled pistachios, toasted and chopped

Nutritional Value: 456 calories per serving

DIRECTIONS

1. Mix 1 teaspoon sugar, rose water, lemon zest, salt and yogurt. Refrigerate the mixture and wait until it is ready for use.
2. In one small saucepan add cardamom pods, water, bay leaves, lemon juice and the rest of the sugar. Cook for 3 minutes and occasionally stir. Add the apricots and cook for 30 more minutes. Take out the apricots and let them cool.
3. Remove the cardamom pods and bay leaves. Boil the syrup over high heat and stir it.
4. Add pistachios on plate. Cut ½ inch opening in each apricot and fill it with the filling. Place the filled apricots on a plate and add syrup all over them.

Fruits and Desserts

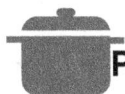 Peaches and Cherries Poached in Spiced Red Wine

COOKING: SERVES: 6

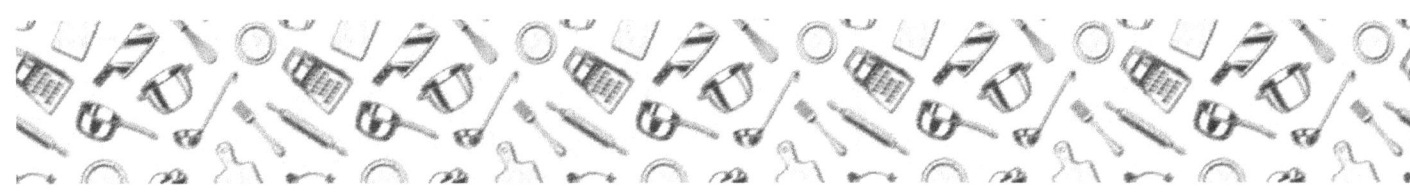

INGREDIENTS

1-pound fresh sweet cherries, pitted and halved
1 pound ripe but firm peaches, sliced ¼ inch thick
½ cinnamon stick
2 whole cloves
2 cups dry red wine
1 cup sugar

Nutritional Value: 258 calories per serving

DIRECTIONS

1. Mix peaches, cherries, cloves and cinnamon sticks in a bowl. Transfer the mixture into a bowl.
2. In small saucepan add red wine and sugar. Wait until it starts boiling and constantly stir until the sugar has dissolved.
3. Pour from the syrup all over the fruit and let it cool in a room temperature.

Fruits and Desserts

 **Pears in Oven with Dried Apricots and Pistachios**

COOKING: 20+ MIN   SERVES: 4

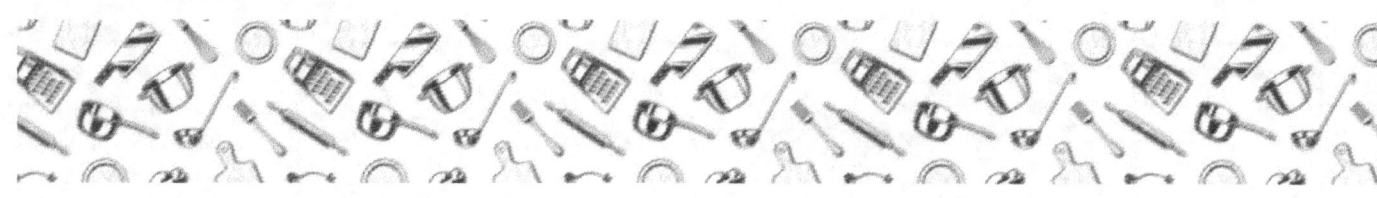

INGREDIENTS

2 tablespoons extra-virgin olive oil
4 ripe but firm Bosc or Bartlett pears
1¼ cups dry white wine
½ cup dried apricots
⅓ cup sugar
¼ teaspoon ground cardamom
⅛ teaspoon salt
1 teaspoon lemon juice
⅓ cup shelled pistachios

Nutritional Value: 258 calories per serving

DIRECTIONS

1. Heat oven up to 450 degrees.
2. In a skillet heat oil over medium-high heat, add the pears side down and cook them for 5 minutes.
3. Place the skillet to oven and roast the pears for 20 minutes.
4. Remove the skilled out of the oven and add the pears into a serving platter.
5. In a skillet over medium heat, add apricots, sugar, cardamom, wine and salt. Cook for 10 minutes with constant stirring. Add the syrup over the pears and sprinkle pistachio crumbs over.

Fruits and Desserts

Apricot Spoon Sweets

COOKING: 40+ MIN

SERVES: 4Cup

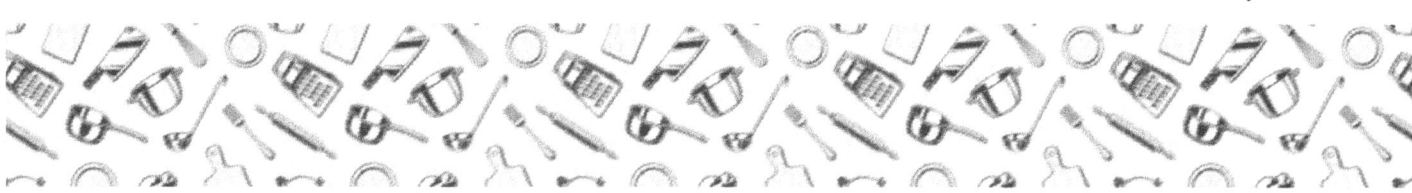

INGREDIENTS

1½ cups sugar
1 cup honey
¾ cup water
1½ pounds ripe but firm apricots, pitted and cut into ½-inch wedges
2 tablespoons lemon juice

Nutritional Value: 313 calories per serving

DIRECTIONS

1. Boil honey, sugar and water over high heat and cook it for 10 minutes with constant stirring.
2. Remove from heat, pour lemon juice and apricots and bring it to boil once again but this time on medium-low heat for 5 minutes.
3. Remove from heat and let it cool.
4. Refrigerate and serve..

Fruits and Desserts

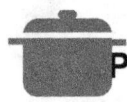 Poached Pears with Lemon, Herbs and White Whine

COOKING: 30+ MIN   SERVES: 8

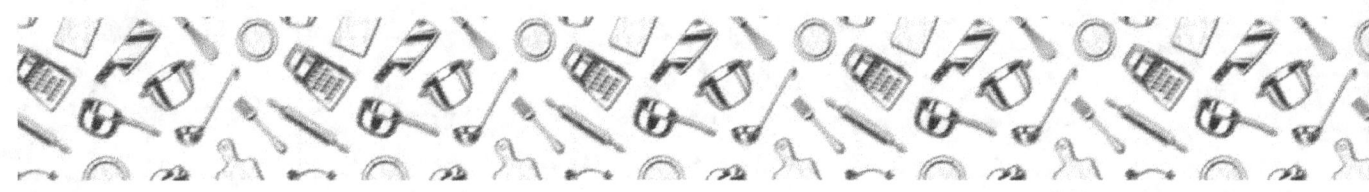

INGREDIENTS

1 vanilla bean
1 bottle dry white wine
¾ cup sugar
6 strips lemon zest
5 sprigs fresh mint
3 sprigs fresh thyme
½ cinnamon stick
⅛ teaspoon salt
6 ripe but firm pears

Nutritional Value: 247 calories per serving

DIRECTIONS

1. Cut the bean in half. Remove the seeds.
2. In large saucepan bring sugar, wine, lemon zest, mint, thyme, cinnamon stick, salt and vanilla seeds to boil over high heat. Cook for 7 minutes.
3. Remove the pod out of the heat, add the pears and return to boil on medium low for 20 minutes. Stir every 5 minutes.
4. Remove the pears in a dish. Simmer the syrup over medium heat for 15 minutes. Add the syrup over the pears..

Fruits and Desserts

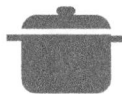 Melon, Plums, and Cherries with Mint and Vanilla

COOKING: 40+ MIN　　　　　　　　　　　　　　　　SERVES: 6

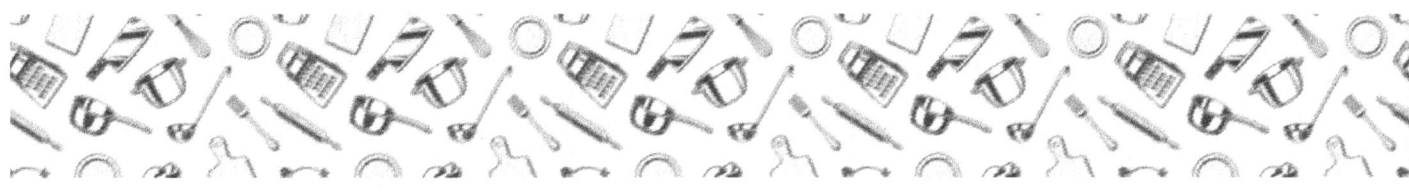

INGREDIENTS

4 teaspoons sugar
1 tablespoon minced fresh mint
3 cups cantaloupe, cut
2 plums
8 ounces fresh sweet cherries
¼ teaspoon vanilla extract
1 tablespoon lime juice, plus extra for seasoning

Nutritional Value: 147 calories per serving

DIRECTIONS

1. In one bowl mix sugar and mint. Press the mixture until the sugar becomes damp. Add plums, cantaloupe, vanilla and cherries. Toss to combine.
2. Leave the mixture for 30 minutes because like that the fruit will release its juices. Add in the lime juice and serve.

Fruits and Desserts

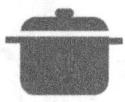

Fruit Mixture with Basil and Pepper

COOKING: 40+ MIN

SERVES: 6

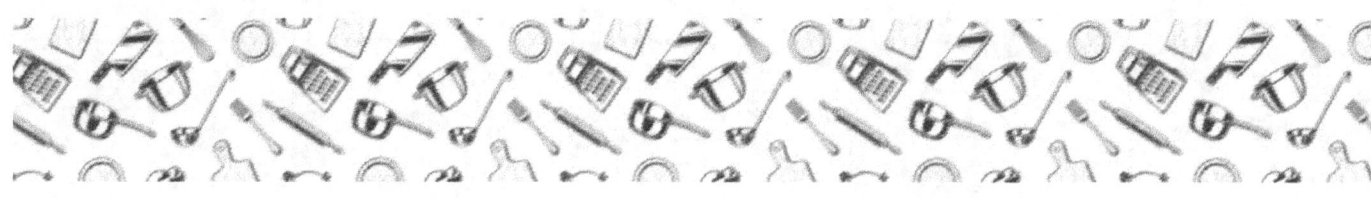

INGREDIENTS

4 teaspoons sugar
2 tablespoons chopped fresh basil
½ teaspoon pepper
3 peaches, halved, pitted, and cut into ½-inch pieces
10 ounces (2 cups) blackberries
10 ounces strawberries, hulled and quartered (2 cups)
1 tablespoon lime juice, plus extra for seasoning

Nutritional Value: 235 calories per serving

DIRECTIONS

1. Mix sugar pepper and basil in a bowl. Press the mixture until the sugar becomes damp. Add blackberries, peaches, strawberries and toss to combine. Leave it on room temperature for at least 30 minutes until the juices are released.
2. Add lime juice over and serve.

Fruits and Desserts

Biscotti with Lemon

COOKING: 40+ MIN

SERVES: 50

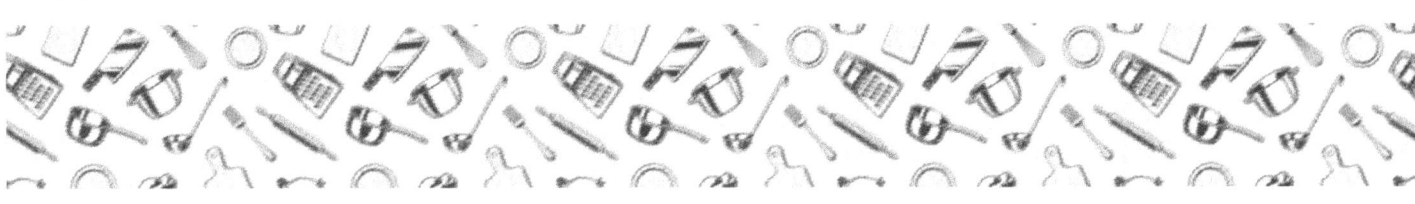

INGREDIENTS

2 cups (10 ounces) all-purpose flour
1 teaspoon baking powder
¼ teaspoon salt
1 cup (7 ounces) sugar
2 large eggs
1 tablespoon grated lemon zest
1 tablespoon anise seeds
¼ teaspoon vanilla extract

Nutritional Value: 325 calories per serving

DIRECTIONS

1. Heat oven to 350 degrees.
2. In a small bowl whisk baking powder, flour and salt. In another large bowl whisk eggs and sugar until you get pale yellow color Add in the lemon zest, anise seeds and vanilla. Stir well until you combine. Add in the flour mixture and stir well once again.
3. Divide the dough. Shape each half into 13 by 2-inch rectangle. Add vegetable oil spray all over the dough. Bake for 35 minutes.
4. Let the loaves cool for 10 minutes and then cut them into ½-inch slices.

Fruits and Desserts

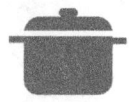

Biscotti with Honey and Lavender

COOKING: 40+ MIN

SERVES: 3

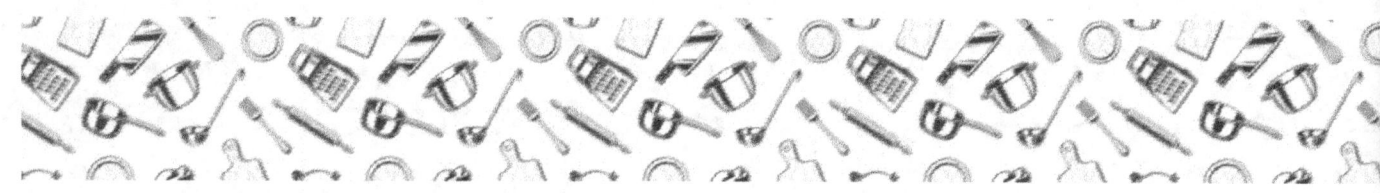

INGREDIENTS

2¼ cups all-purpose flour
1 teaspoon baking powder
½ teaspoon baking soda
¼ teaspoon salt
3 large eggs
3 tablespoons honey
2 tablespoons grated orange zest
1 tablespoon dried lavender
½ teaspoon vanilla extract

Nutritional Value: 233 calories per serving

DIRECTIONS

1. Heat oven to 350 degrees.
2. In a small bowl whisk baking powder, flour, baking soda and salt. In another large bowl whisk eggs and sugar until you get pale yellow color. Add in orange zest, lavender, honey and vanilla. Stir well until you combine. Add in the flour mixture and stir well once again.
3. Divide the dough. Shape each half into 13 by 2-inch rectangle. Add vegetable oil spray all over the dough. Bake for 35 minutes.
4. Let the loaves cool for 10 minutes and then cut them into ½-inch slices.

Fruits and Desserts

Lemon Rice Pudding from Greece

COOKING:

SERVES: 8

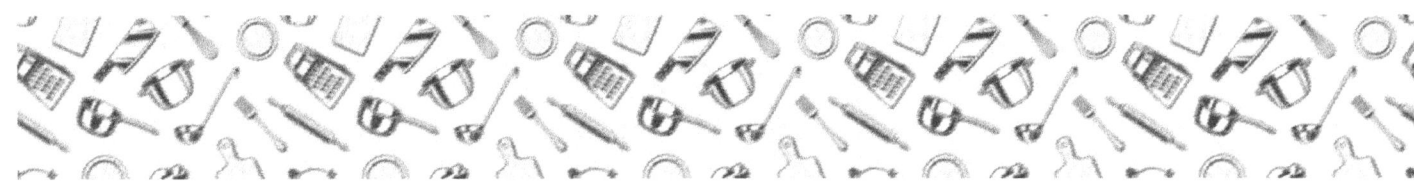

INGREDIENTS

2 cups water
1 cup Arborio rice
½ teaspoon salt
1 vanilla bean
4½ cups whole milk, plus extra as needed
½ cup sugar
½ cinnamon stick
2 bay leaves
2 teaspoons grated lemon zest

DIRECTIONS

1. In a large saucepan over medium-high heat bring water to boil. Add in the rice and salt. Reduce the heat and simmer for 20 minutes.
2. Take the vanilla bean and cut it in half. Remove the seeds and add it into the rice. Stir and add the milk, sugar, cinnamon stick, and bay leaves. Increase the heat and cook it for 45 more minutes.
3. Remove the bay leaves, cinnamon stick and vanilla bean. Add in the lemon zest. Let it cool for at least 2 hours. Stir the pudding and serve..

Fruits and Desserts

Raspberry Sorbet

COOKING: 15+ MIN

SERVES: 8

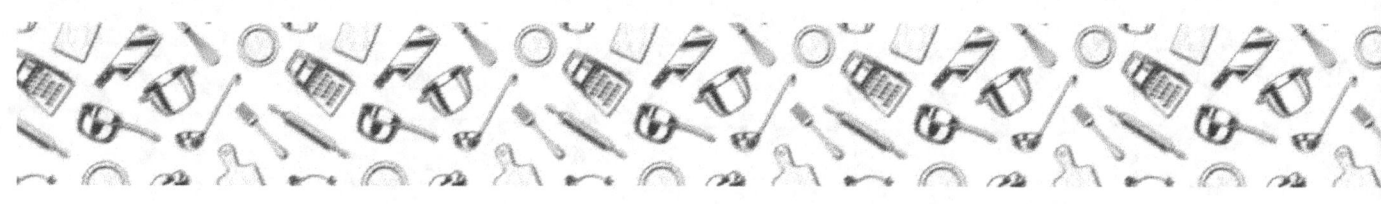

INGREDIENTS

1 cup water
1 teaspoon low fruit pectin
⅛ teaspoon salt
1¼ pounds fresh or frozen raspberries
½ cup (3½ ounces) plus 2 tablespoons sugar
¼ cup light corn syrup

Nutritional Value: 258 calories per serving

DIRECTIONS

1. Over medium high heat, in a saucepan add water, pectin and salt. Cook it with constant stirring for at least 5 minutes. Remove it from heat and let it cool for at least 10 minutes.
2. In a blender add raspberries, corn syrup, sugar and cooled water mixture. Blend it for at least 30 seconds and then strain the mixture. In a small bowl add 1 cup of the mixture and place the rest of the mixture in a large bowl. Cover with plastic wrap and place both mixtures in refrigerator. Wait until they are completely.

Fruits and Desserts

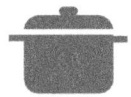

Lemon Ice with Mint

COOKING: 15+ MIN

SERVES: 8

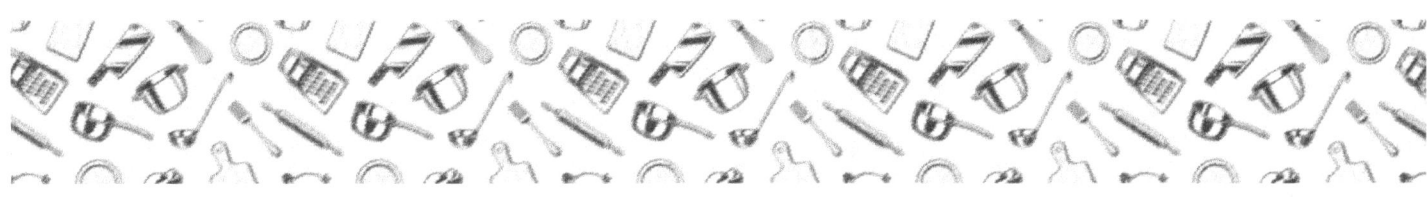

INGREDIENTS

2¼ cups water
1 cup lemon juice
1 cup sugar
2 tablespoons vodka
⅛ teaspoon salt
10 mint leaves

Nutritional Value: 324 calories per serving

DIRECTIONS

1. In a bowl place all the ingredients and constantly whisk until you dissolve the sugar. Add the mixture over 2 ice cube trays and freeze it.
2. You need to wait for approximately 20 hours until the mixture freezes. Then, remove it out of the freezer and place the cubes in a food processor. Pulse and serve.

Fruits and Desserts

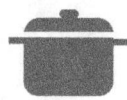 

Orange Ice with Mint

COOKING: 15+ MIN   SERVES: 8

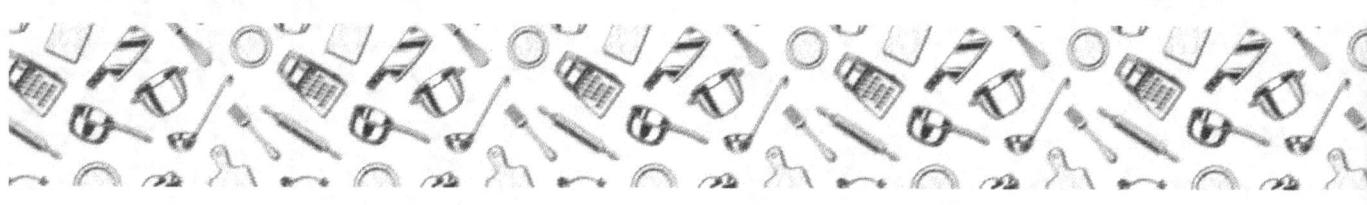

INGREDIENTS

2¼ cups water
1 cup orange juice
1 cup sugar
2 tablespoons vodka
⅛ teaspoon salt
10 mint leaves

Nutritional Value: 244 calories per serving

DIRECTIONS

1. In a bowl place all the ingredients and constantly whisk until you dissolve the sugar. Add the mixture over 2 ice cube trays and freeze it.
2. You need to wait for approximately 20 hours until the mixture freezes. Then, remove it out of the freezer and place the cubes in a food processor. Pulse and serve.

Fruits and Desserts

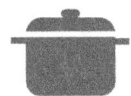

Vanilla Baked Pears

COOKING: 30 MIN

SERVES: 30

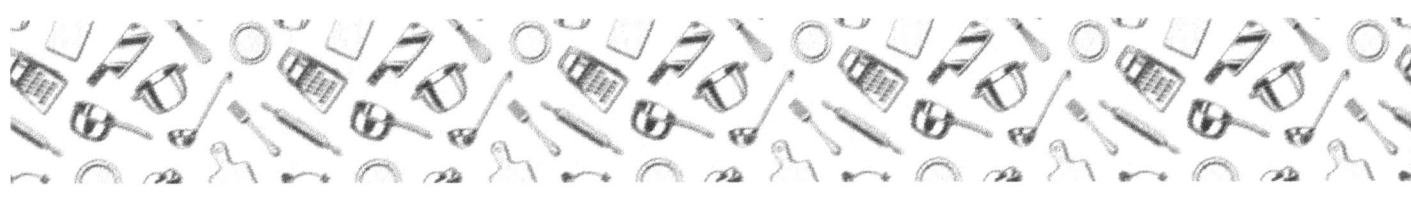

INGREDIENTS

4 pears
1 cup maple syrup
1 teaspoon cinnamon
1 teaspoon vanilla extract
Greek Yogurt

Nutritional Value: 103 calories per serving

DIRECTIONS

1. Warm up the oven to reach 375° Fahrenheit.
2. Slice each of the pears into halves. Slice off a small sliver on the underneath side so it will lay flat.
3. Remove the seeds from the core and place on a baking sheet with the face side up and sprinkle with the cinnamon.
4. Whisk the syrup and vanilla. Drizzle over the pears. Save 2 tablespoons for the garnishing.
5. Place in the oven and bake for 25 minutes or until softened.
6. When done, place in the serving dishes and drizzle with the rest of the maple syrup mixture.
7. Serve with a dollop of yogurt.

Fruits and Desserts

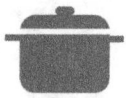

Dark Chocolate Fruit Kebabs

COOKING: 20 MIN

SERVES: 6

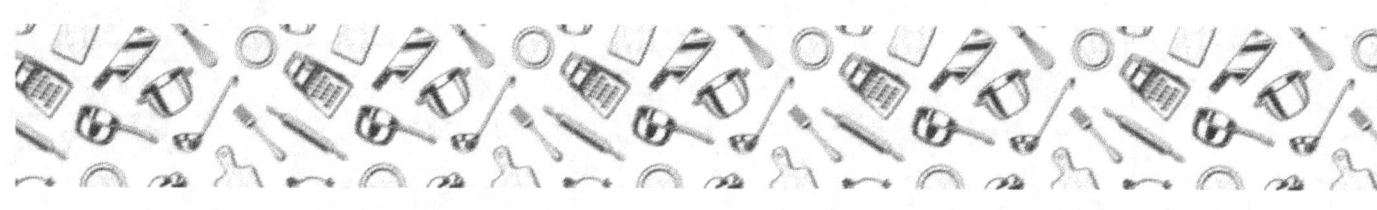

INGREDIENTS

12 strawberries
24 grapes
12 cherries
24 blueberries
8 oz. dark chocolate

Nutritional Value: 254 calories per serving

DIRECTIONS

1. Prepare a rimmed baking sheet with a layer of parchment paper. Lay out six 12-inch skewers. Prepare the skewers with the fruit - alternating each flavor.
2. Use a microwave-safe dish to heat the chocolate on high for one minute. Stir to melt the chocolate.
3. Add the melted chocolate to a plastic sandwich bag and twist a corner. Snip the corner off of the bag to use as a pipe. Squeeze the bag to drizzle the chocolate over the kebabs.
4. Arrange the sheet in the freezer to chill for 20 minutes before serving.

Fruits and Desserts

Butter Cookies

COOKING: 20 MIN   SERVES: 8

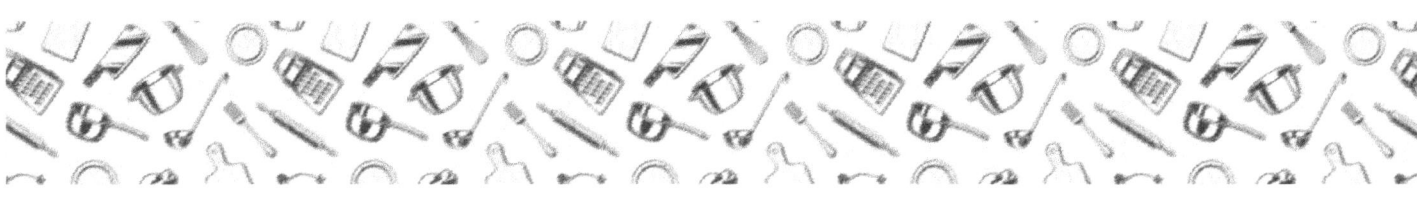

INGREDIENTS

1 cup butter, softened
3/4 cup white raw honey
1 egg
1/2 teaspoon vanilla extract
1/2 teaspoon almond extract
2 1/4 cups all-purpose flour
1/2 cup confectioners' raw honey for rolling

Nutritional Value: 254 calories per serving

DIRECTIONS

1. Preheat the oven to 400 degrees F (200 degrees C). Grease cookie sheets.
2. In a medium bowl, cream together the butter, raw honey and egg until smooth. Stir in the vanilla and almond extracts. Blend in the flour to form a dough. you may have to knead by hand at the end. Take about a teaspoon of dough at a time and roll into balls, logs or 'S' shapes. Place cookies 1 to 2 inches apart onto the prepared cookie sheets.
3. Bake for 10 minutes in the preheated oven, or until lightly browned and firm. Allow cookies to cool completely before dusting with confectioners' raw honey.

Fruits and Desserts

Strawberry Tiramisu

COOKING: 20 MIN

SERVES: 8

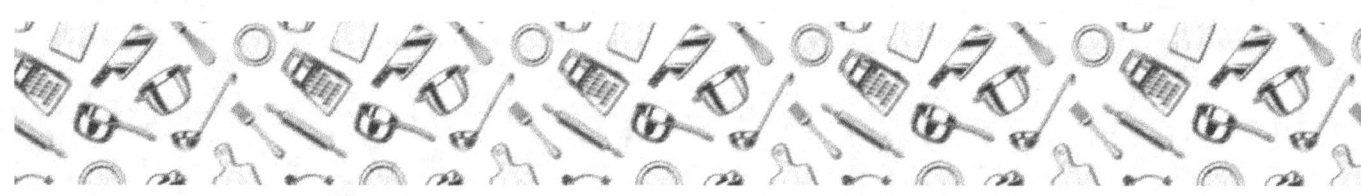

INGREDIENTS

1 (8 ounce) package Cream Cheese, softened
3 1/2 cups cold milk
2 (3.4 ounce) packages Instant Pudding
2 (3 ounce) packages ladyfingers, split
1 (6 ounce) tub Strawberry Creme, thawed
2 1/2 cups sliced fresh strawberries
2 squares Semi-Sweet Chocolate, grated

Nutritional Value: 215 calories per serving

DIRECTIONS

1. Beat cream cheese in large bowl with mixer until creamy. Gradually add milk, beating until well blended. Add dry pudding mixes; beat on low speed 1 min. or until well blended.
2. Cover bottom of 13x9-inch pan with half the ladyfingers; top with layers of half each of the pudding mixture, COOL WHIP DIPS and berries. Repeat all layers.
3. Refrigerate 3 hours. Sprinkle with chocolate.

Fruits and Desserts

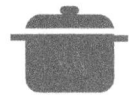

Spicy Biscotti

COOKING: 40+ MIN SERVES: 10+

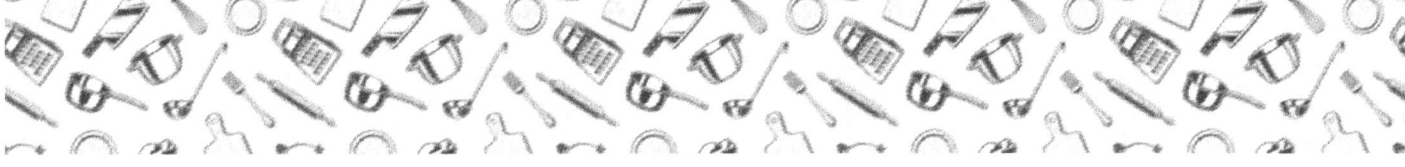

INGREDIENTS

2¼ cups all-purpose flour
1 teaspoon baking powder
½ teaspoon baking soda
½ teaspoon ground cloves
½ teaspoon ground cinnamon
¼ teaspoon ground ginger
¼ teaspoon salt
¼ teaspoon ground white pepper
1 cup sugar
2 large eggs plus 2 large yolks
½ teaspoon vanilla extract

Nutritional Value: 258 calories per serving

DIRECTIONS

1. Heat oven to 350 degrees.
2. In a small bowl add flour, baking powder, baking soda, cloves, cinnamon, ginger, salt and pepper. In another, large bowl add sugar, eggs, egg yolks and whisk it. Add in the vanilla.
3. Divide the dough. Shape each half into 13 by 2-inch rectangle. Add vegetable oil spray all over the dough. Bake for 35 minutes.
4. Let the loaves cool for 10 minutes and then cut them into ½-inch slices.

Fruits and Desserts

Honey-Glazed Peaches with Hazelnuts

COOKING: 40+ MIN   SERVES: 4

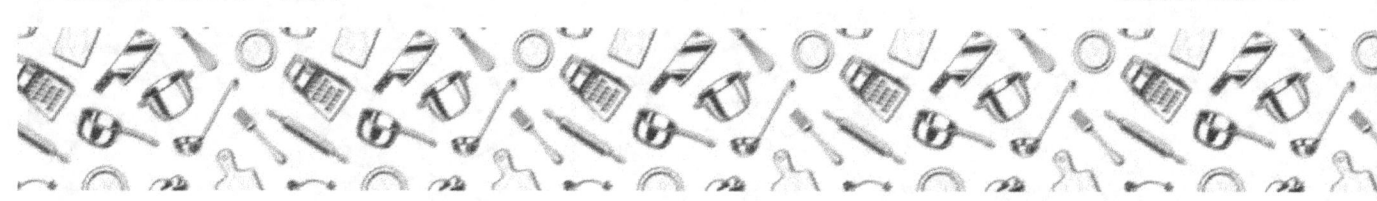

INGREDIENTS

2 tablespoons lemon juice
1 tablespoon sugar
¼ teaspoon salt
6 ripe but firm peaches, peeled, halved, and pitted
⅓ cup water
¼ cup honey
1 tablespoon extra-virgin olive oil
¼ cup hazelnuts

Nutritional Value: 313 calories per serving

DIRECTIONS

1. Mix sugar, salt and lemon juice in a bowl. Add the peaches and toss to combine. Make sure that each side is covered with the sugar mixture.
2. Place them in a skillet and add the rest from the sugar mixture. Add water and broil the peaches for 15 minutes.
3. In another bowl mix honey and oil and use the microwave to dissolve the honey. Pour from the honey all over the peach mixture and return them to broil for another 8 minutes.
4. Remove the skillet from the oven and serve.

Fruits and Desserts

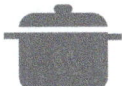 **Plums in Oven with Dried Cherries and Almonds**

COOKING: SERVES: 8

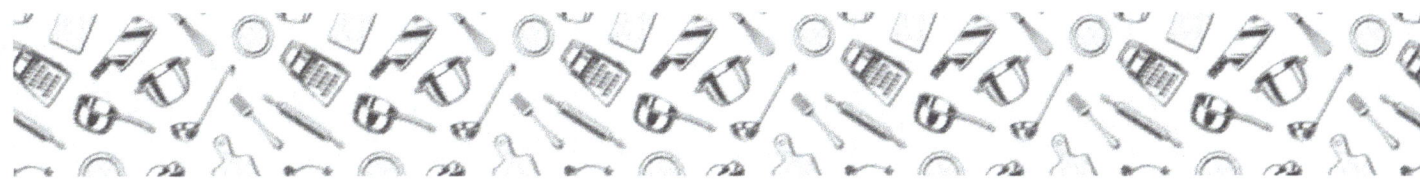

INGREDIENTS

- 4 unpeeled plums
- ½ cup dried cherries
- ⅓ cup sugar
- 1 teaspoon lemon juice
- ¼ teaspoon cinnamon
- 1/3 cup sliced almonds

DIRECTIONS

1. Heat oven up to 450 degrees.
2. In a skillet heat oil over medium-high heat, add the plums side down and cook them for 5 minutes.
3. Place the skillet to oven and roast the apples for 20 minutes.
4. Remove the skilled out of the oven and add the pears into a serving platter.
5. In a skillet over medium heat, add cherries, sugar, cardamom, red wine and salt. Cook for 10 minutes with constant stirring. Add the syrup over the plums and sprinkle almond crumbs over.

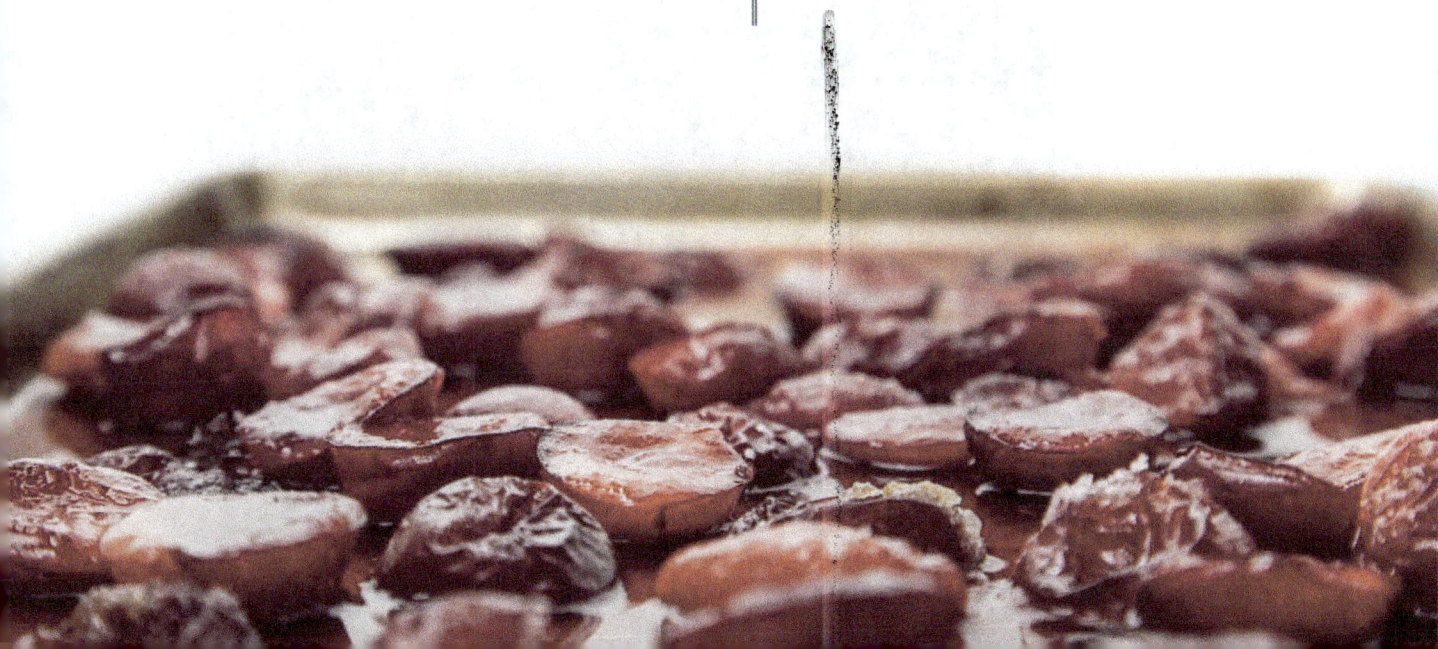

Fruits and Desserts

Balsamic Strawberries

COOKING: 40+ MIN

SERVES: 6

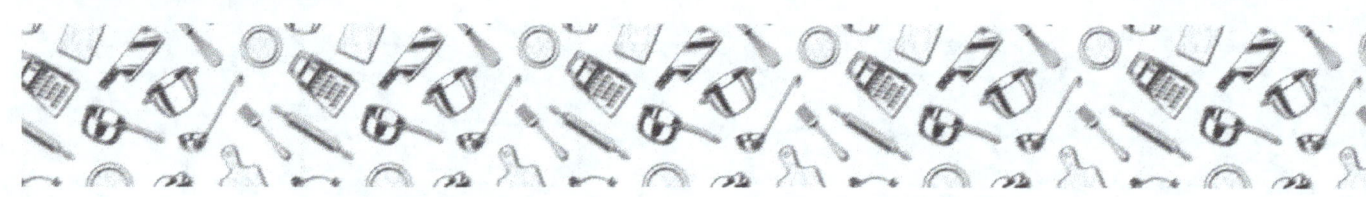

INGREDIENTS

⅓ cup balsamic vinegar
2 pounds strawberries
¼ inch thick (5 cups)
2 teaspoons granulated sugar
½ teaspoon lemon juice
¼ cup pepper

Nutritional Value: 362 calories per serving

DIRECTIONS

1. In a saucepan add sugar, vinegar and lemon juice. Cook it over medium heat for 5 minutes. Remove the syrup into a small bowl.
2. Add the strawberries in a bowl and spread over sugar and pepper. Pour the syrup all over the strawberries and toss to combine.

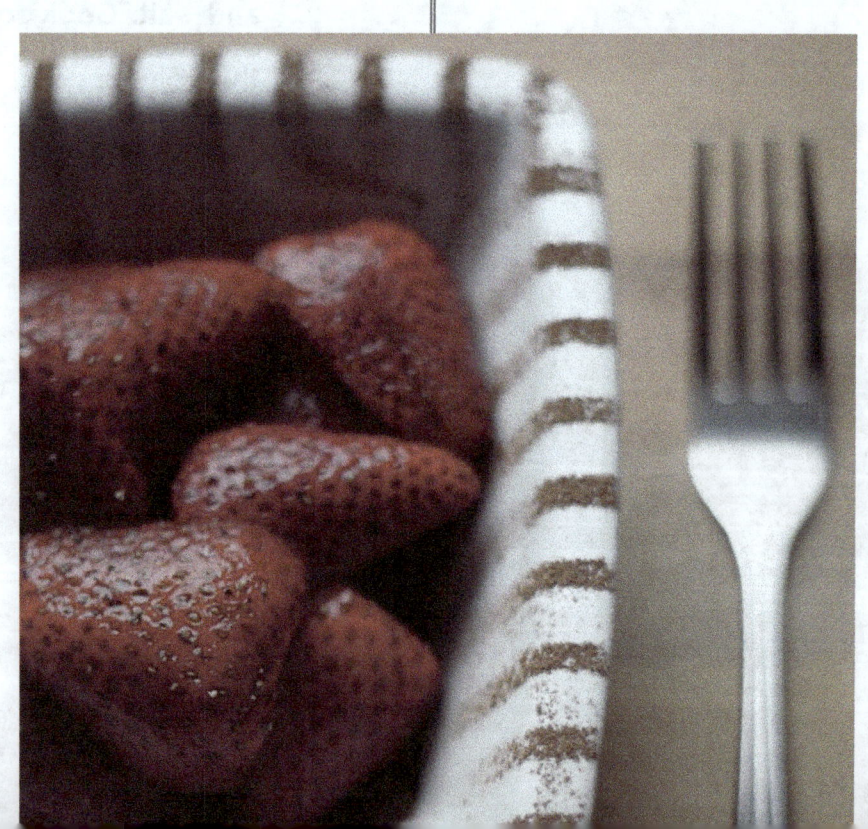

Fruits and Desserts

Pignoli

COOKING: 15+ MIN

SERVES: 18 Cookies

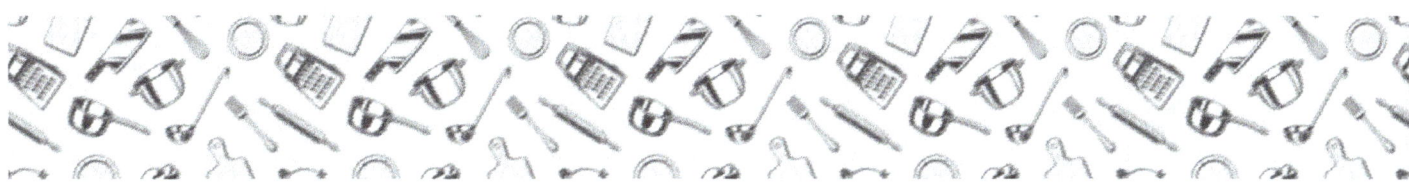

INGREDIENTS

1⅔ cups slivered almonds
1⅓ cups (9⅓ ounces) sugar
2 large egg whites
1 cup pine nuts

Nutritional Value: 214 calories per serving

DIRECTIONS

1. Heat oven to 375 degrees.
2. In a food processor add almonds and sugar. Process the ingredients until you get smooth mixture. Add egg whites and start processing again. Make sure that the final mixture looks smooth. Transfer it into a bowl.
3. With one tablespoon scoop mixture out of the dough, roll into balls, add pine nuts to coat and place it on a baking pan. Repeat the procedure with each dough scoop.
4. Bake the cookies for 15 minutes. Remove them, let them cool and serve.

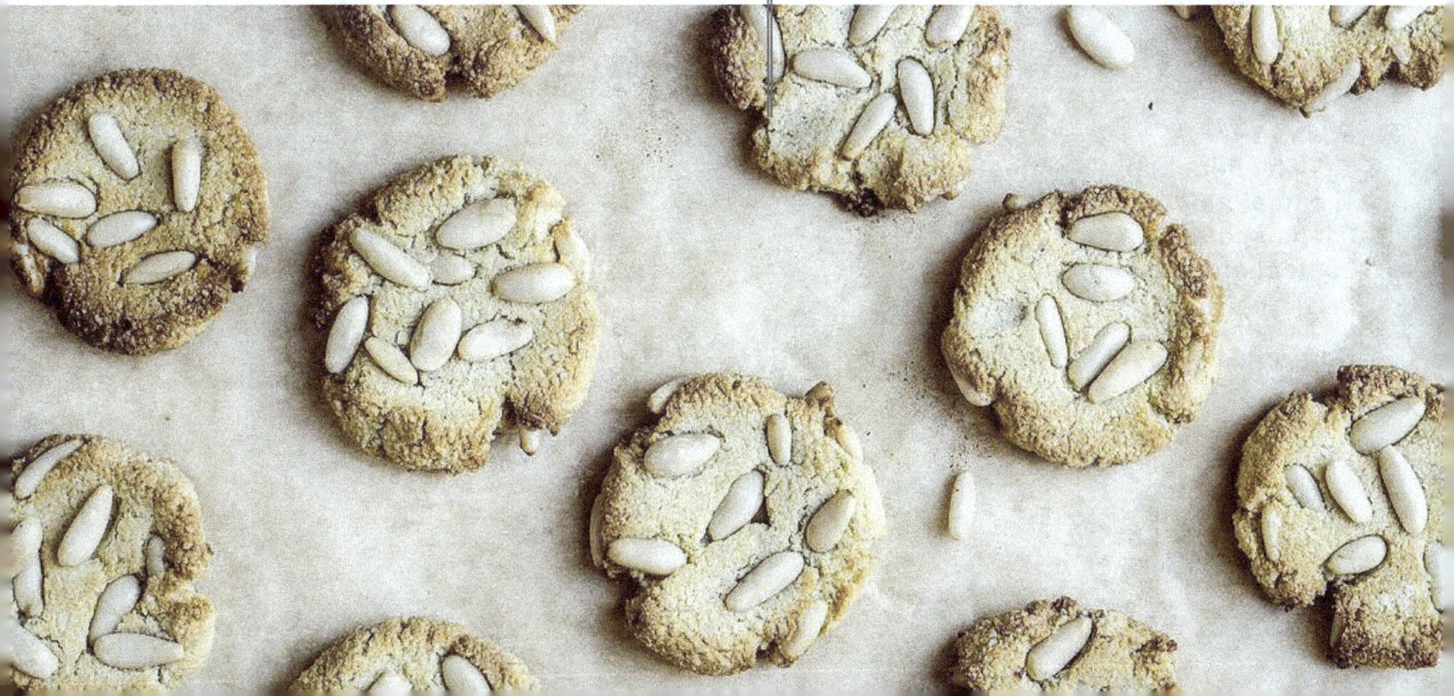

Fruits and Desserts

Fig Phyllo Cookies

COOKING: 15+ MIN   SERVES: 24 Cookies

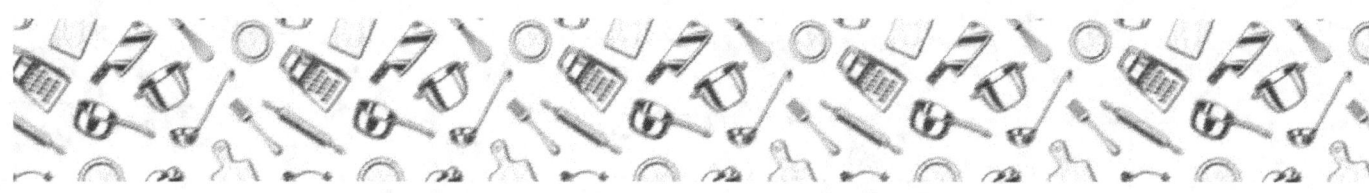

INGREDIENTS

Sugar syrup
¼ cup granulated sugar
2 tablespoons water
2 tablespoons honey
2 (2-inch) strips orange zest plus
2 tablespoons juice

Fig filling
1½ cups (9 ounces) dried figs, stemmed and halved
¾ cup water
½ cup granulated sugar
1 teaspoon orange zest
½ teaspoon anise seeds
½ cup walnuts, toasted and chopped coarse
1 tablespoon dry sherry

Pastry
6 (14 by 9-inch) phyllo sheets, thawed
¼ cup extra-virgin olive oil
2 tablespoons confectioners' sugar

Nutritional Value: 452 calories per serving

DIRECTIONS

1. *Sugar syrup:* In a saucepan add every ingredient and cook it over medium-high heat. Cook it for two minutes or cook it at least until you dissolve the sugar. Remove the zest and insert the syrup into a bowl.
2. *Fig filling:* Heat water, sugar, orange zest, anise seeds and figs in a saucepan over medium heat. Cook the ingredients for five minutes. Add the ingredients into a food processor and process them for 15 seconds.
3. *Pastry*: Heat oven to 375 degrees. Put a baking sheet and parchment paper on the baking pan. Add one phyllo sheet and brush it with oil. Immediately dust it with one teaspoon sugar. Repeat the procedure with two more phyllo sheets. At the bottom edge of each phyllo add from the filling but remember, leave 1 ½ inch border. Then, fold the bottom edge over the filling and roll the phyllo. To be more specific, form a cylinder and then cut it into 12 different pieces. Repeat the procedure with the rest 3 phyllo sheets.
4. Bake the cookies for 20 minutes until light golden brown. Remove them from oven and drizzle syrup over them.

Fruits and Desserts

Almond Cake

COOKING: 15+ MIN   SERVES: 12

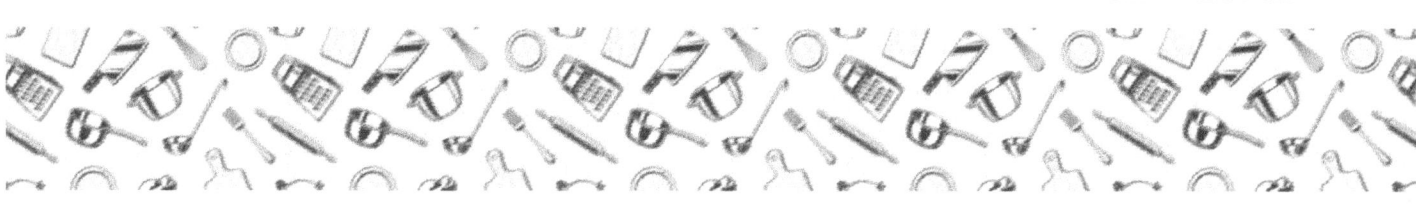

INGREDIENTS

1½ cups plus ⅓ cup blanched sliced almonds, toasted
¾ cup (3¾ ounces) all-purpose flour
¾ teaspoon salt
¼ teaspoon baking powder
⅛ teaspoon baking soda
4 large eggs
1¼ cups (8¾ ounces) plus 2 tablespoons sugar
1 tablespoon plus ½ teaspoon grated lemon zest (2 lemons)
¾ teaspoon almond extract
½ cup extra-virgin olive oil

Nutritional Value: 321 calories per serving

DIRECTIONS

1. Heat oven too 300 degrees. Take one cake pan and grease it.
2. In a food processor pulse 1 ½ cups almonds, salt, baking powder, flour and baking soda. Pulse the ingredients until you get finely ground almonds. Transfer the mixture into a bowl.
3. In the same processor add eggs, 1 ¼ cups sugar, 1 tablespoon lemon zest, and almond extract. Pulse it for 30 seconds. Add in the almond mixture and process for additional 10 seconds.
4. Place the batter into a pan. In a bowl add the remaining 2 tablespoons of sugar and lemon zest. Mix well and sprinkle over the cake.
5. Bake the cake for approximately 65 minutes. Rotate the pan after 40 minutes.

Fruits and Desserts

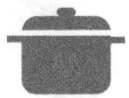 

Polenta Cake

COOKING: 15+ MIN   SERVES: 12

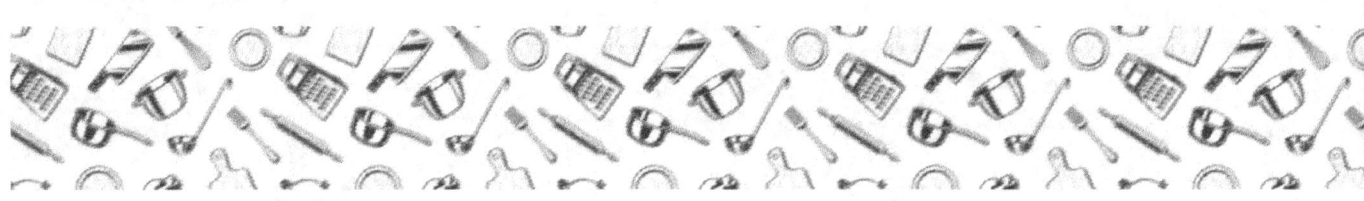

INGREDIENTS

1½ cups (8¼ ounces) instant polenta
1½ cups whole milk
3 large eggs
1 cup (7 ounces) granulated sugar
6 tablespoons extra-virgin olive oil
2 oranges plus
2 teaspoons grated orange zest
⅓ cup (2⅓ ounces) packed brown sugar
2 teaspoons cornstarch
1 teaspoon baking powder
½ teaspoon baking soda
2 teaspoons vanilla extract
Salt
1 cup (5 ounces) all-purpose flour

Nutritional Value: 258 calories per serving

DIRECTIONS

1. Heat oven to 350 degrees. In rimmed baking sheet spread the polenta and toast it for 10 minutes. Place it into a large bowl. Add milk and orange zest and let it like that for 10 minutes. Use your hands and break the polenta into crumbs. Put it aside.
2. Take a cake pan and grease it. Mix brown sugar, cornstarch, and 1/8 tablespoon salt in small bowl. Sprinkle the bottom of the pan. Remove the peel and slice the oranges into 1/8-inch slices. Put the orange slices in one single layer over the sugar mixture.
3. In a bowl mix baking powder, flour, baking soda and ½ teaspoon salt. In another bowl beat eggs and granulated sugar by using stand mixer. Lower the speed and add oil and vanilla. Beat until you combine them and then add polenta crumbs. Continue to beat until you combine them. Add flour mixture next and continue to beat until you perfectly combine the mixture.
4. Pour the batter over the oranges and bake the cake for 60 minutes.

Fruits and Desserts

Olive Oil–Yogurt Cake

COOKING: 15+ MIN   SERVES: 12

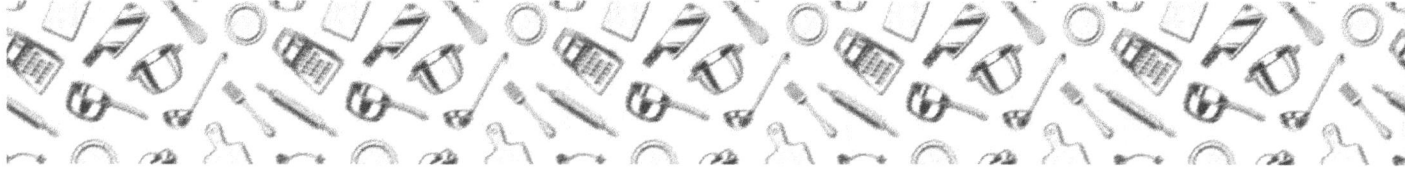

INGREDIENTS

3 cups (15 ounces) all-purpose flour
1 tablespoon baking powder
1 teaspoon salt
1¼ cups (8¾ ounces) granulated sugar
4 large eggs
1¼ cups extra-virgin olive oil
1 cup plain whole-milk yogurt
Glaze
2–3 tablespoons lemon juice
1 tablespoon plain whole-milk yogurt
2 cups (8 ounces) confectioners' sugar

Nutritional Value: 326 calories per serving

DIRECTIONS

1. *Cake* – Heat oven too 350 degrees. Take a nonstick baking pan and grease it. In a bowl mix baking powder, flour and salt. In another bowl mix sugar and eggs. Stir until you dissolve the sugar. Add in the oil and yogurt. Transfer the batter into the pan and bake the cake for 45 minutes or until it gets golden brown color.
2. *Lemon glaze* – In a bowl whisk yogurt, two tablespoons of lemon juice, and confectioners' sugar. Pour from the mixture over the cake.

Fruits and Desserts

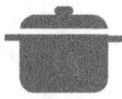

Lemon Mousse with Blueberry Sauce

COOKING: 15+ MIN

SERVES: 6

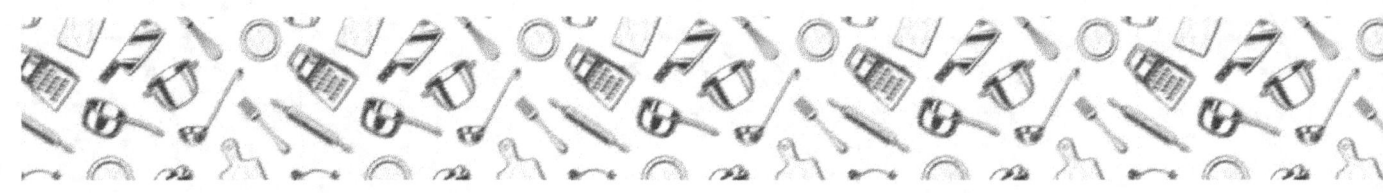

INGREDIENTS

Sauce:
4 ounces (¾ cup) blueberries
2 tablespoons sugar
2 tablespoons water
Pinch salt
Mousse:
¾ teaspoon unflavored gelatin
3 tablespoons water
½ cup whole Greek yogurt
¼ cup heavy cream
1½ teaspoons grated lemon zest plus
3 tablespoons juice
1 teaspoon vanilla extract
⅛ teaspoon salt
3 large egg whites
¼ teaspoon cream of tartar
6 tablespoons (2⅔ ounces) sugar

Nutritional Value: 258 calories per serving

DIRECTIONS

1. *Sauce*: In a saucepan bring blueberries, water, salt and sugar to boil over medium heat. Cook for at least 5 minutes. Transfer the mixture into a blender and blend it for 30 seconds. Remove the blended mixture out of the blender, place it in six different ramekins and refrigerate for 20 minutes.
2. *Mousse*: Add gelatin over water in one bowl and let it like that for at least five minutes.
3. In another bowl add heavy cream, yogurt, lemon zest, juice, vanilla and salt.
4. In third bowl mix cream of tartar, egg whites and sugar with stand mixer. Transfer it in a saucepan over medium-heat and cook it for 10 minutes.
5. Add the dissolved gelatin and transfer the mixture in a bowl once again. Use the stand mixer and whip over medium-high speed for 7 minutes. Add in the yogurt mixture and continue to whip.
6. Place from the mousse over the chilled remekins.

Fruits and Desserts

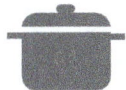

Baklava

COOKING: 150+ MIN

SERVES: 30 Pieces

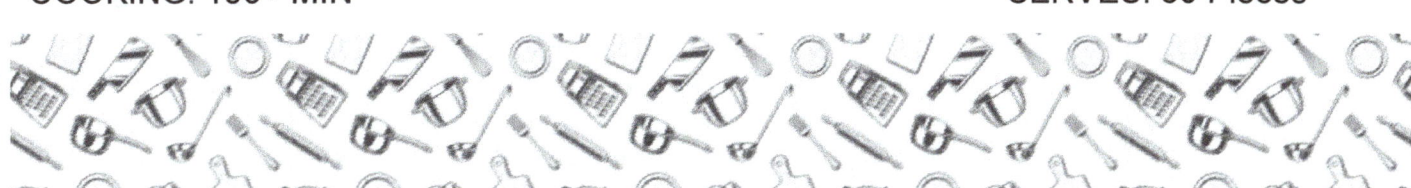

INGREDIENTS

Sugar syrup
1¼ cups (8¾ ounces) sugar
¾ cup water
⅓ cup honey 3 (2-inch) strips lemon zest plus 1 tablespoon juice
1 cinnamon stick
5 whole cloves
⅛ teaspoon salt

Filling
1¾ cups slivered almonds
1 cup walnuts
2 tablespoons sugar
1¼ teaspoons ground cinnamon
¼ teaspoon ground cloves
⅛ teaspoon salt

Pastry
5 tablespoons extra-virgin olive oil
1-pound (14 by 9-inch) phyllo, thawed

Nutritional Value: 362 calories per serving

DIRECTIONS

1. *Sugar syrup* – In a saucepan add all the ingredients over medium-high heat. Cook it until you dissolve the sugar, approximately five minutes. Take it out of the heat, transfer it into a measuring cup and let it cool.
2. *Nut Filling* – In a food processor, add the almonds and pulse for at least 20 times. Transfer them into a bowl and then repeat the procedure with the walnuts. Mix the ingredients together and toss to combine them well. Add sugar, cloves, salt and cinnamon and toss once again.
3. *Pastry* – Heat oven to 300 degrees. Grease the baking pan. Lay one phyllo sheet at the bottom and brush oil over it. Repeat the procedure with 7 more sheets. Brush each with oil and make sure that you have 8 layers.
4. Take one cup of nut filling and spread evenly over the sheets. Cover with 6 more phyllo sheets (make sure each has oil between). Add one cup of the feeling once again and cover with sheets once again. Add 8 more sheets, brush each with oil and on the final layer add two tablespoons of oil.
5. Cur the baklava into diamonds. Put it in the oven and bake it for 1 ½ hours.
6. Right after removing the baklava from the oven pour the syrup over the cut lines. Let the baklava cool for at least 3 hours, covered with aluminum foil. It is recommended that you need to wait for at least 8 hours before consumption.

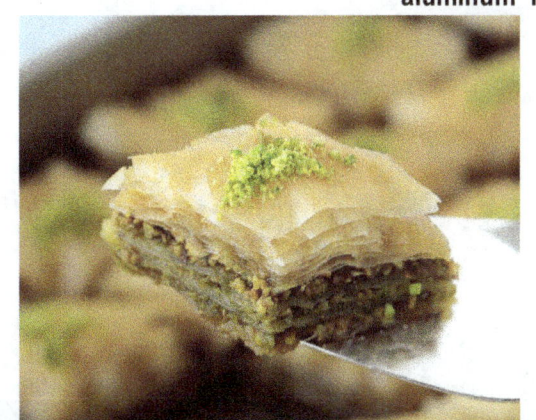

Fruits and Desserts

 **Lemon Yogurt Mousse with Strawberry Sauce**

COOKING: 15+ MIN   SERVES: 6

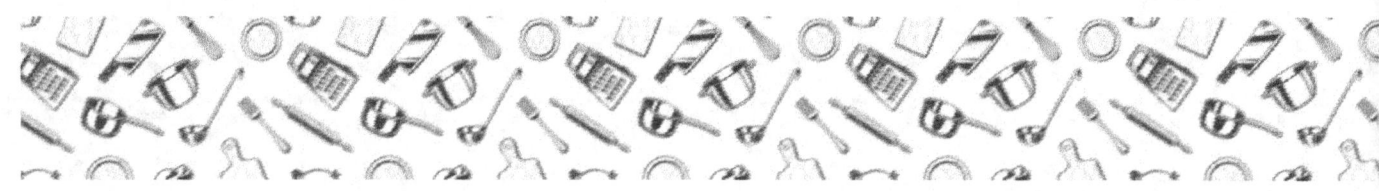

INGREDIENTS

Sauce:
4 ounces (¾ cup) strawberries
2 tablespoons sugar
2 tablespoons water
Pinch salt
Mousse:
¾ teaspoon unflavored gelatin
3 tablespoons water
½ cup whole Greek yogurt
¼ cup heavy cream
1½ teaspoons grated lemon zest plus
3 tablespoons juice
1 teaspoon vanilla extract
⅛ teaspoon salt
3 large egg whites
¼ teaspoon cream of tartar
6 tablespoons (2⅔ ounces) sugar

Nutritional Value: 365 calories per serving

DIRECTIONS

1. Sauce: In a saucepan bring strawberries, water, salt and sugar to boil over medium heat. Cook for at least 5 minutes. Transfer the mixture into a blender and blend it for 30 seconds. Remove the blended mixture out of the blender, place it in six different ramekins and refrigerate for 20 minutes.
2. Mousse: Add gelatin over water in one bowl and let it like that for at least five minutes.
3. In another bowl add heavy cream, yogurt, lemon zest, juice, vanilla and salt.
4. In third bowl mix cream of tartar, egg whites and sugar with stand mixer. Transfer it in a saucepan over medium-heat and cook it for 10 minutes.
5. Add the dissolved gelatin and transfer the mixture in a bowl once again. Use the stand mixer and whip over medium-high speed for 7 minutes. Add in the yogurt mixture and continue to whip.
6. Place from the mousse over the chilled ramekins.

Fruits and Desserts

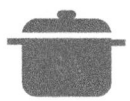

Almonds and Dates Semolina Pudding

COOKING: 15+ MIN

SERVES: 8

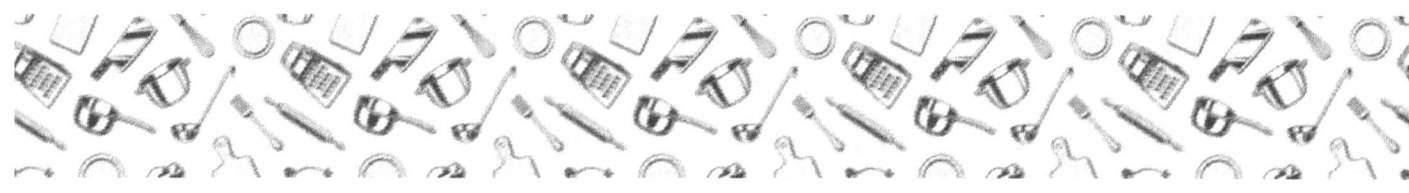

INGREDIENTS

1 tablespoon extra-virgin olive oil
¾ cup fine semolina flour
4½ cups whole milk, plus extra as needed
½ cup sugar
½ teaspoon ground cardamom
⅛ teaspoon saffron threads, crumbled
⅛ teaspoon salt
½ cup slivered almonds, toasted and chopped
3 ounces pitted dates, sliced thin

Nutritional Value: 214 calories per serving

DIRECTIONS

1. Over medium heat, in a skillet cook the semolina. Cook and stir it for at least five minutes.
2. In one large saucepan, over medium heat, add milk, sugar, saffron, salt and cardamom. Whisk constantly and add the semolina. Cook until the mixture is combined for 3 minutes. Remove it from heat and let it cool for 30 minutes.
3. Add in the pudding and add milk if necessary when it comes to the consistency. Add almonds and dates over.

Fruits and Desserts

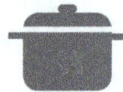

Lemon Ice

COOKING: 15+ MIN

SERVES: 8

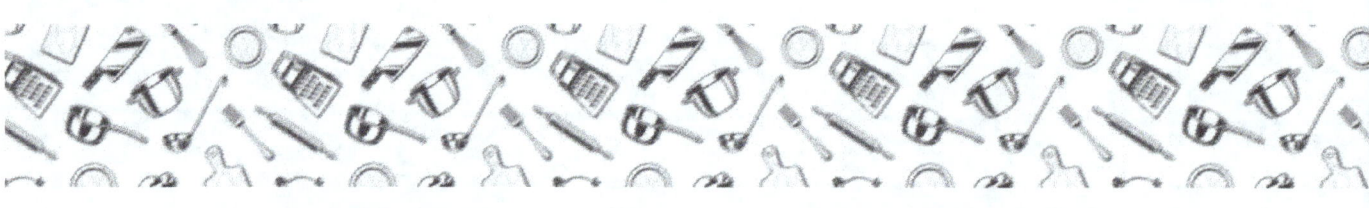

INGREDIENTS

- 2¼ cups water
- 1 cup lemon juice
- 1 cup sugar
- 2 tablespoons vodka
- ⅛ teaspoon salt

Nutritional Value: 694 calories per serving

DIRECTIONS

1. In a bowl place all the ingredients and constantly whisk until you dissolve the sugar. Add the mixture over 2 ice cube trays and freeze it.
2. You need to wait for approximately 20 hours until the mixture freezes. Then, remove it out of the freezer and place the cubes in a food processor. Pulse and serve.

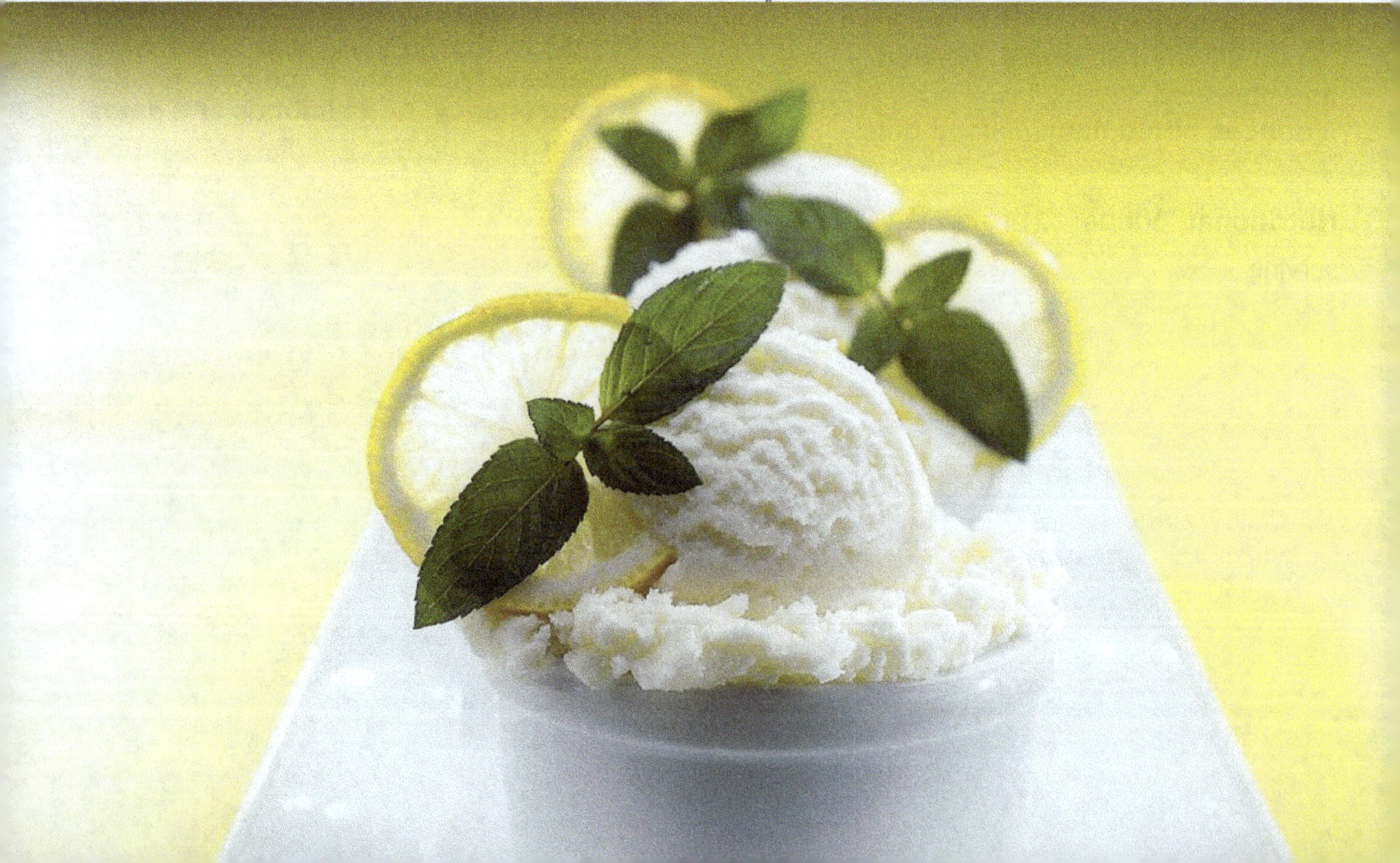

Fruits and Desserts

 **Cake for New Year's**

COOKING: 50+ MIN   SERVES: 8

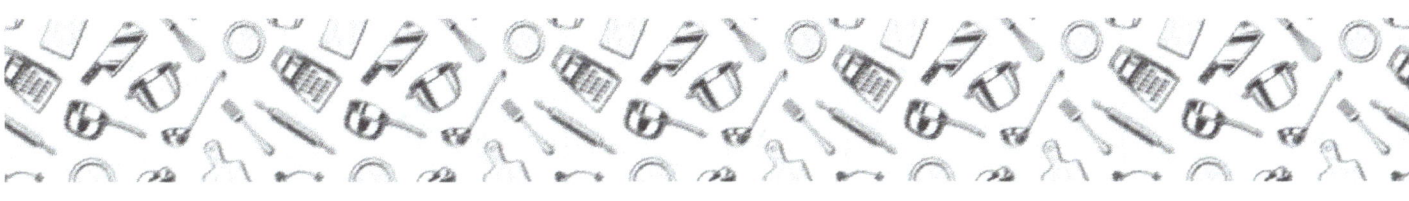

INGREDIENTS

1 cup butter
2 cups white raw honey
3 cups all-purpose flour
6 eggs
2 teaspoons baking powder
1 cup warm milk
1/2 teaspoon baking soda
tablespoon fresh lemon juice
1/4 cup blanched slivered almonds
3 tablespoons white raw honey

Nutritional Value: 358 calories per serving

DIRECTIONS

1. Preheat oven to 350 degrees F (175 degrees C). Generously grease a 10-inch round cake pan.
2. In a medium bowl, cream the butter and raw honey together until light. Stir in the flour and mix until the mixture is mealy. Add the eggs one at a time, mixing well after each addition. Mix the baking powder and milk, add to the egg mixture, mix well. Then Mix the lemon juice and baking soda, stir into the batter. Pour into the prepared cake pan.
3. Bake for 20 minutes in the preheated oven. Remove and sprinkle the nuts and raw honey over the cake, then return it to the oven for 20 to 30 additional minutes, until cake springs back to the touch. Gently slice a small hole in the cake and place a quarter in the hole. Try to cover the hole with raw honey. Cool cake on a rack for 10 minutes before inverting onto a plate.
4. Serve cake warm. Each person in the family gets a slice starting with the youngest. The person who gets the quarter in their piece, gets good luck for the whole year!

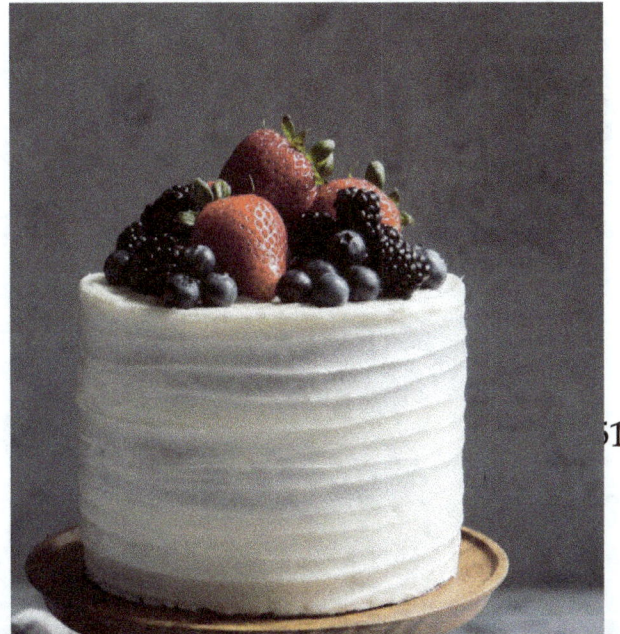

Fruits and Desserts

Banana Sour Cream Bread

COOKING: 25 MIN   SERVES: 8

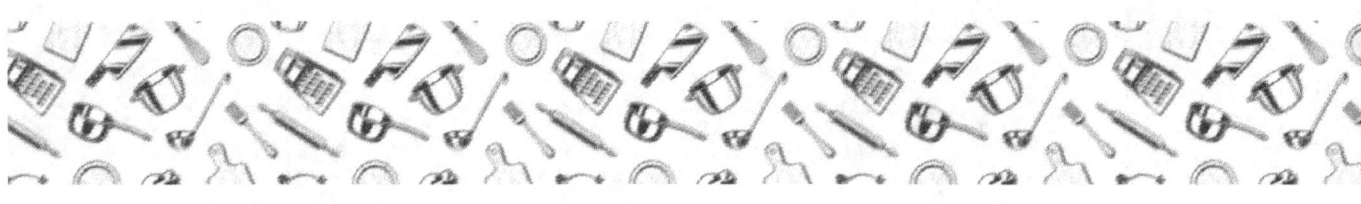

INGREDIENTS

1 cup honey
1 teaspoon cinnamon
1 butter
3 cup raw honey
3 eggs
6 bananas
16 oz sour cream
2 teaspoons vanilla
 3 teaspoons cinnamon
3 teaspoons baking soda
4 cups flour
1 cup chopped walnuts

Nutritional Value: 236 calories per serving

DIRECTIONS

1. Warm up the oven to reach 300°Fahrenheit. Grease the loaf pans.
2. Sift the raw honey and one teaspoon of the cinnamon. Dust the pan with the mixture.
3. Cream the butter with the rest of the raw honey. Mash the bananas with the eggs and Mix with the cinnamon, vanilla, sour cream, salt, baking soda, and the flour. Toss in the nuts last.
4. Pour the mixture into the pans. Bake for 1 hour. Test for doneness with a toothpick in the center. It's done when it comes out clean.

Fruits and Desserts

 **Pears Filled with Almonds**

COOKING: 50 MIN					SERVES: 4

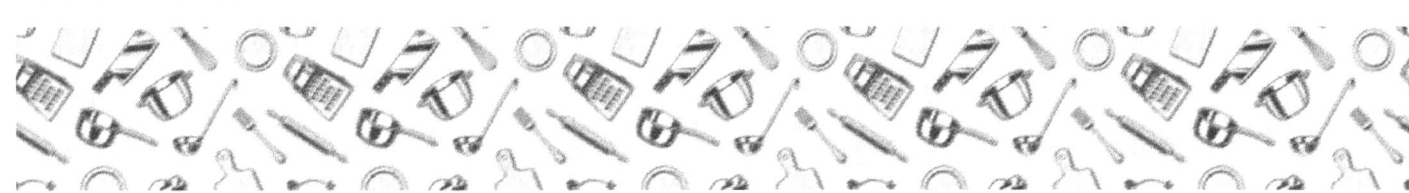

INGREDIENTS

6 medium pears, peeled, halved, and cored
1 1/2 cups water
1/3 cup white grape juice
1/2 cup finely chopped toasted almonds
2 tablespoons brown sugar
1/8 teaspoon almond extract

Nutritional Value: 333 calories per serving

DIRECTIONS

1. Place pears cut side down, in an ungreased 13-in. x 9-in. x 2-in baking dish. Combine water and grape juice; pour over pears.
2. Cover and bake at 350 degrees F for 35-45 minutes or until tender. Turn the pears over. Combine almonds, sugar and extract; mix well. Spoon into pear cavities. Bake, uncovered, for 5 minutes. Serve warm.

Smoothies

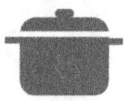

Mango Pear Smoothie

COOKING: SERVES: 1

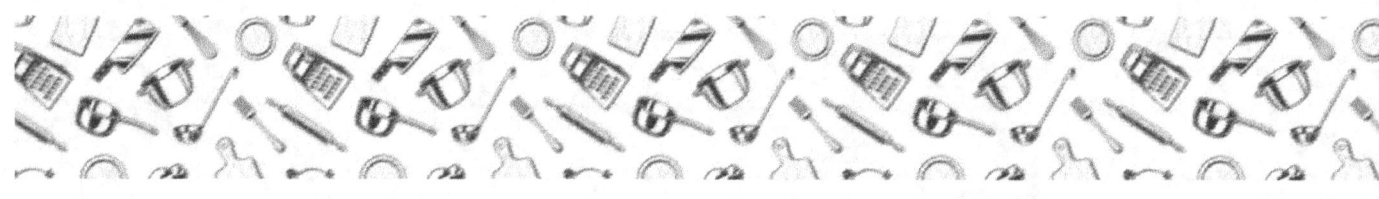

INGREDIENTS

1 cup Greek yogurt
2 ice cubes
1 cup mango
1 cup kale
1 pear

Nutritional Value: 125 calories per serving

DIRECTIONS

1. Mix each of the Ingredients in a blender.
2. Mix well until thickened and smooth.
3. Serve in a chilled glass.

Smoothies

 **Lemon and Strawberries Smoothie**

COOKING: SERVES: 1

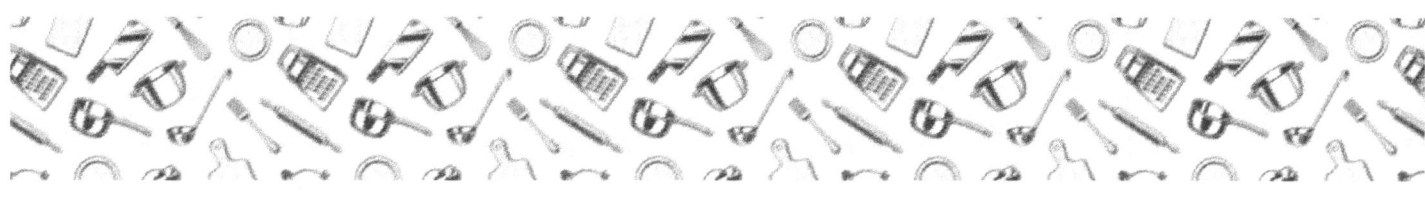

INGREDIENTS

1 cup nonfat vanilla yogurt
1/2 cup orange juice
1 1/2 cup strawberries
1/2 cup crushed ice
1 T. lemon juice
1/2 tsp. lemon zest

Nutritional Value: 125 calories per serving

DIRECTIONS

1. Combine all in blender until smooth.

Smoothies

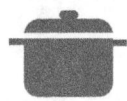 Orange-Pineapple Smoothie

COOKING: SERVES: 1

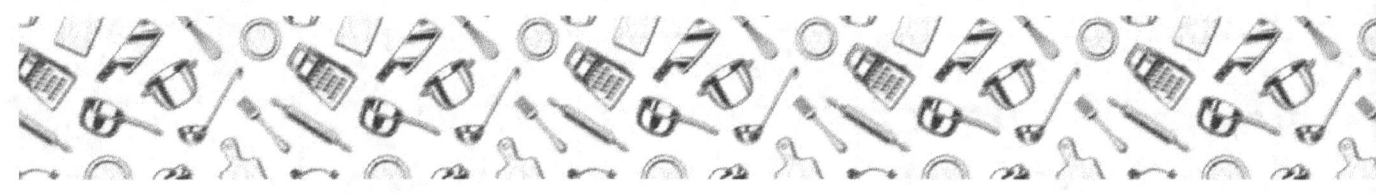

INGREDIENTS

1 (8 ounce) can canned pineapple chunks, undrained
1 (6 ounce) can froze orange juice concentrate
1 cup white rum
2 tablespoons sugar
1 tablespoon lime juice 1 tray ice
4 maraschino cherries, garnish

Nutritional Value: 254 calories per serving

DIRECTIONS

1. In a blender, Mix pineapple, orange juice concentrate with juice, rum, sugar, lime juice and ice cubes. Blend until smooth. Pour into glasses, garnish with cherries, and serve.

Smoothies

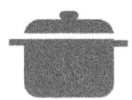

Pineapple Orange Smoothie

COOKING:

SERVES: 1

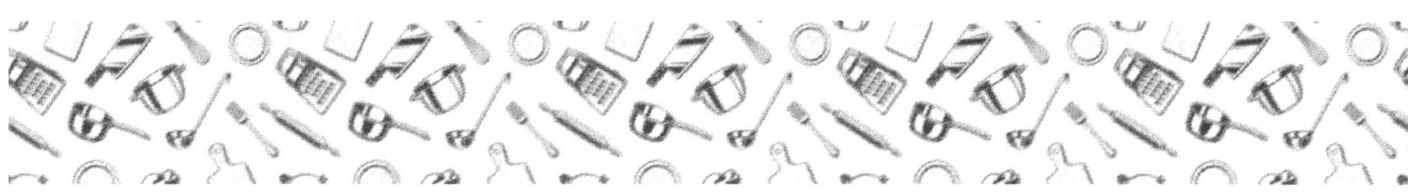

INGREDIENTS

1 cup pineapple juice
1 cup orange juice
1/2 frozen banana (chunks)
1 cup pineapple sherbet
1 1/2 cups frozen mango slices

Nutritional Value: 470 calories per serving

DIRECTIONS

1. Pour all liquid Ingredients into the blender. Add all frozen Ingredients. Blend at MIX setting for 30 seconds then blend at Smooth setting until smooth. While the machine is running, move the stir stick around counterclockwise to aid mixing. Serve immediately. Each recipe serves 3-5.

Smoothies

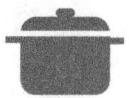

Peach Smoothie

COOKING: SERVES: 1

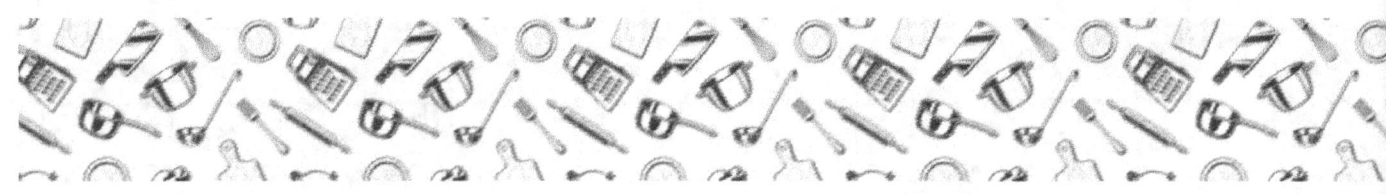

INGREDIENTS

1 cup sliced peaches
4 cubes ice (optional)
1/4 teaspoon ground nutmeg
1/2 teaspoon vanilla extract
1/2 teaspoon honey
2 teaspoons wheat germ
1 tablespoon rolled oats 1 cup vanilla soymilk

Nutritional Value: 144 calories per serving

DIRECTIONS

1. Place the peaches, ice, nutmeg, vanilla extract, honey, wheat germ, oats, and soymilk into a blender. Cover, and puree until smooth.
2. Pour into glasses to serve.

Smoothies

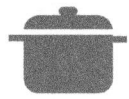 **Pear and Strawberries Smoothie**

COOKING: SERVES: 1

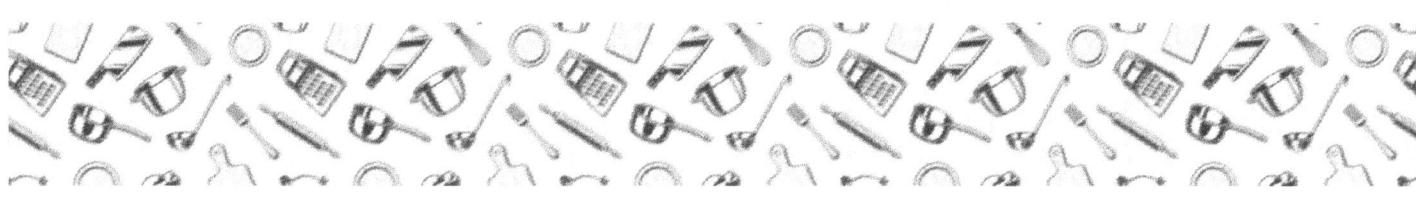

INGREDIENTS

1/2 cup ice
1 Asian pear, cored and cubed
2 large strawberries, hulled
2/3 cup vanilla fat-free yogurt
1/4 cup fat-free milk
2 teaspoons white sugar

Nutritional Value: 244 calories per serving

DIRECTIONS

1. Place the ice, Asian pear, strawberries, yogurt, milk, and sugar into a blender, blend until smooth.

Smoothies

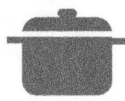

Strawberry R. Smoothie

COOKING: SERVES: 1

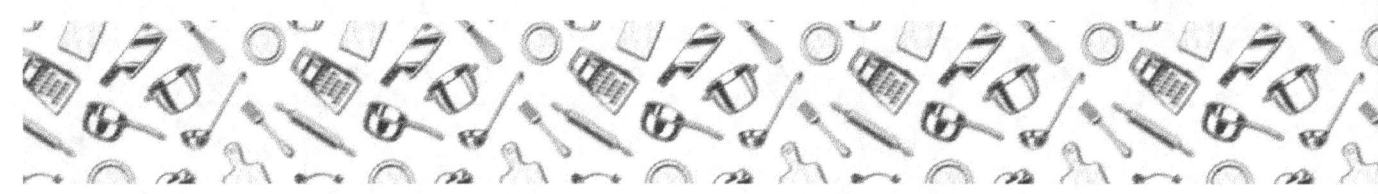

INGREDIENTS

- 1 cup strawberries
- 1 stalk chopped rhubarb
- 2 tablespoons honey
- 3 ice cubes
- 1 tablespoon cinnamon
- 5 cups yogurt

1. **Nutritional Value**: 295 calories per serving

DIRECTIONS

Pour water into a small saucepan and add the rhubarb. Boil for 3 minutes before draining and adding to a blender.
2. Prepare the rest of the fixings and add to the blender along with the honey, yogurt, cinnamon, and ice.
3. Blend well until creamy smooth, serving a chilled glass.

Smoothies

Peanut Butter Smoothie

COOKING:

SERVES: 1

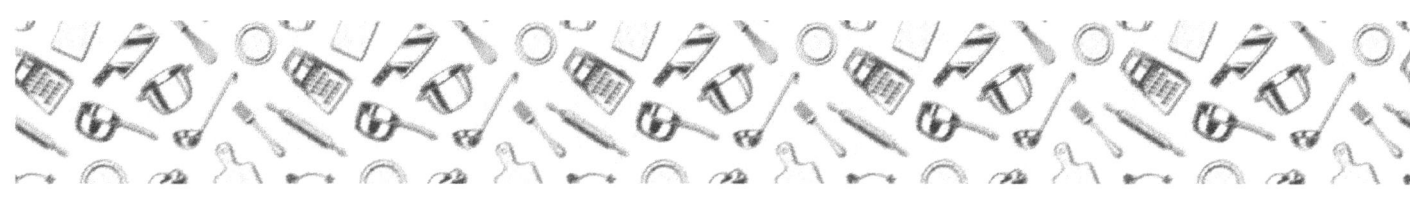

INGREDIENTS

1/2 cup soymilk
1/2 cup silken tofu
1/3 cup creamy peanut butter
2 bananas frozen
2 tablespoons chocolate syrup

Nutritional Value: 255 calories per serving

DIRECTIONS

1. Combine soymilk, tofu, and peanut butter in blender. Add bananas, chocolate syrup, and any ice cubes if desired. Blend until smooth. Serves

Smoothies

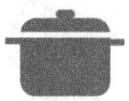

Nectarine Smoothie

COOKING: SERVES: 1

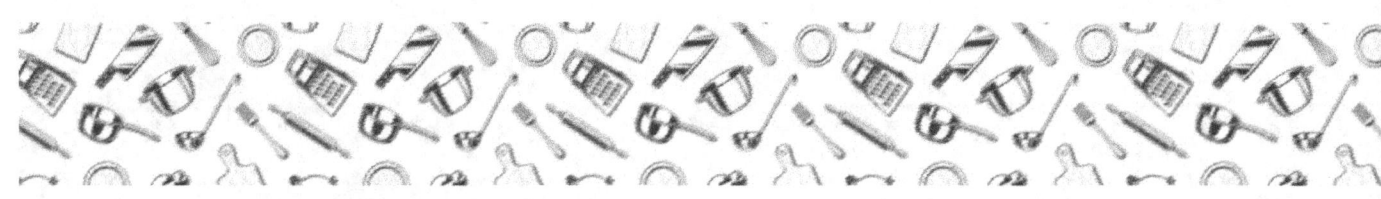

INGREDIENTS

1. 1 nectarine, pitted
2. 3/4 cup strawberries, hulled
3. 3/4 cup blueberries, rinsed and drained
4. 1/3 cup nonfat dry milk powder
5. 1 cup crushed ice
6.
7. **Nutritional Value**: 236 calories per serving

DIRECTIONS

1. In a blender combine nectarine, strawberries, blueberries, milk powder and crushed ice. Blend until smooth. pour into glasses and serve.

Smoothies

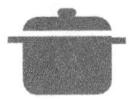

Pineapple Ginger Smoothie

COOKING:

SERVES: 1

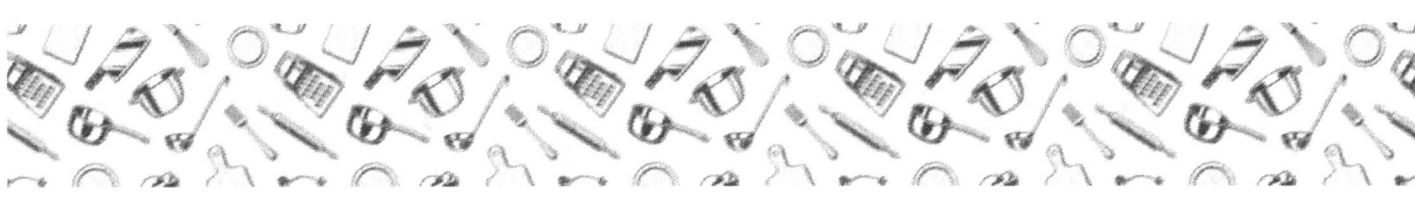

INGREDIENTS

1/2 cup Orange juice
1/4 cup Pineapple juice
1/2 Banana
1/4 Ginger root
Ice cubes

Nutritional Value: 214 calories per serving

DIRECTIONS

1. Blend all until smooth.

Smoothies

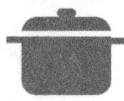 Orange and Strawberry Smoothie

COOKING: SERVES: 1

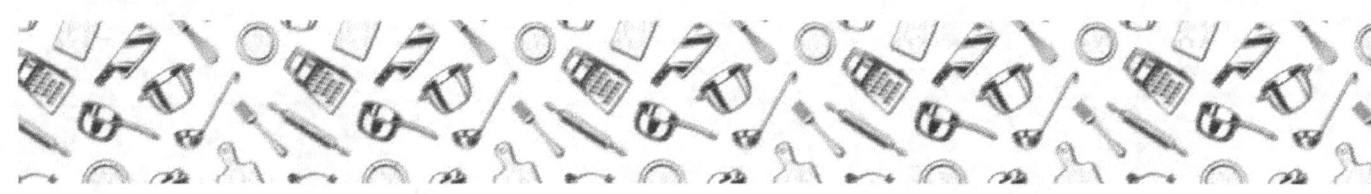

INGREDIENTS

1 cup chopped fresh strawberries
1 cup orange juice
10 cubes ice
1 tablespoon sugar

Nutritional Value: 144 calories per serving

DIRECTIONS

1. In a blender, combine strawberries, orange juice, ice cubes and sugar. Blend until smooth. Pour into glasses and serve.

Smoothies

Melon Mint Smoothie

COOKING:

SERVES: 1

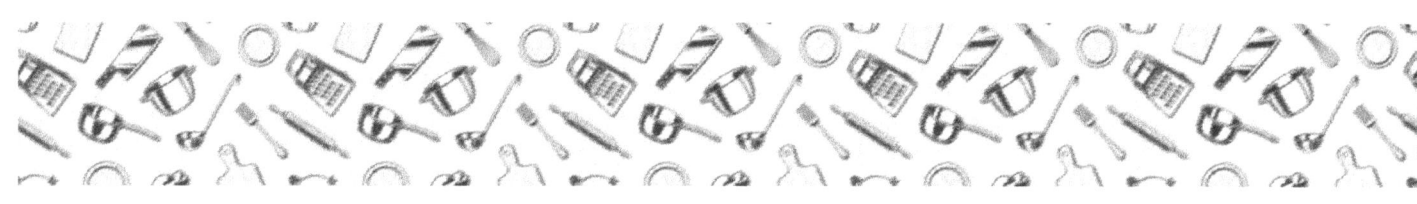

INGREDIENTS

2 cups diced cantaloupe
1 cup diced honeydew melon
1 cup diced seedless watermelon
1/2 cup passion fruit or mango juice
1 tablespoon lime juice
2 teaspoons honey
10 fresh mint leaves
3 ice cubes

Nutritional Value: 211 calories per serving

DIRECTIONS

1. Combine all Ingredients in blender and whip until smooth.

Smoothies

Pineapple Berry Smoothie

COOKING:

SERVES: 1

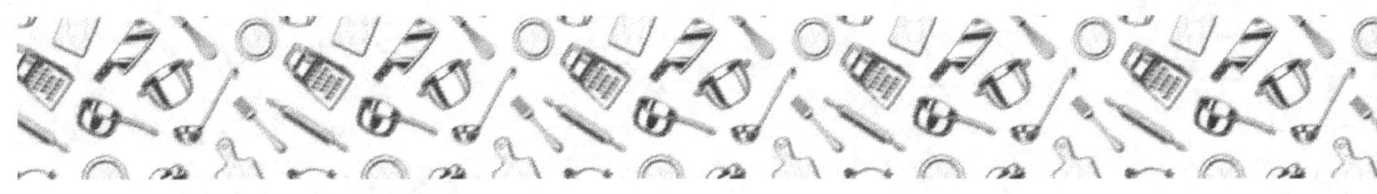

INGREDIENTS

1 cup orange juice
1/4 cup pineapple juice
2 pineapple rings (Dole pineapple slices)
6 fresh strawberries
12-15 frozen raspberries
8-10 frozen boysenberries
12-15 frozen blueberries
3 oz. non-fat yogurt, any flavor (about half a container of Yoplait)
Ice (however much
you prefer for consistency)

Nutritional Value: 214 calories per serving

DIRECTIONS

1. Put all Ingredients into blender. Blend well until smoothie consistency is reached!

Smoothies

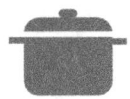 **Papaya Smoothie**

COOKING: SERVES: 1

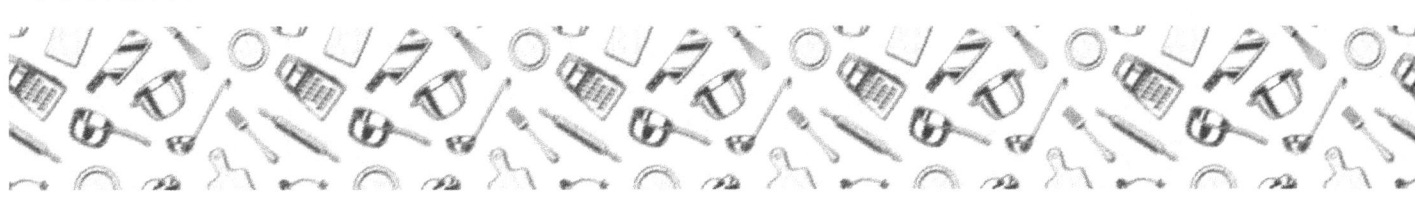

INGREDIENTS

1 frozen banana (freezing it makes the drink super cold without diluting it with ice)
1/2 fresh papaya
10-12 raspberries (fresh or frozen)
1/2 c water or fruit juice
1 tbsp toasted wheat germ (optional)

Nutritional Value: 214 calories per serving

DIRECTIONS

1. Puree in blender 30-45 seconds. makes about sixteen delicious, filling, vegan, nutritious ounces.

Smoothies

Coconut Smoothie

COOKING: SERVES: 1

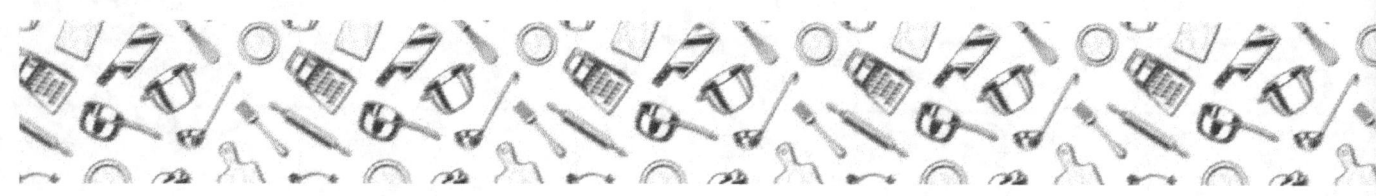

INGREDIENTS

1/4 cup apple juice
1 pinch grated coconut or 1 T. coconut milk
1/2 banana
1/4 teaspoon fresh ginger root peeled
2 small ice cubes

Nutritional Value: 156 calories per serving

DIRECTIONS

1. Put all Ingredients into blender.
2. Blend until smoothie consistency is reached!

Smoothies

Pistachio Smoothie

COOKING: SERVES: 1

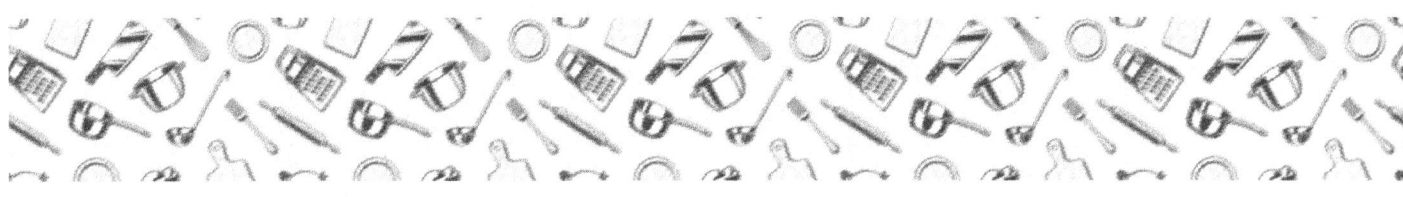

INGREDIENTS

1 container plain nonfat yogurt
2-3 oz pistachio instant pudding mix
1 ripe banana
1/4 c skim milk
handful or more of crushed ice

Nutritional Value: 369 calories per serving

DIRECTIONS

1. Put all Ingredients into blender. Blend until smoothie consistency is reached!

Smoothies

Oatmeal Smoothie

COOKING: SERVES: 1

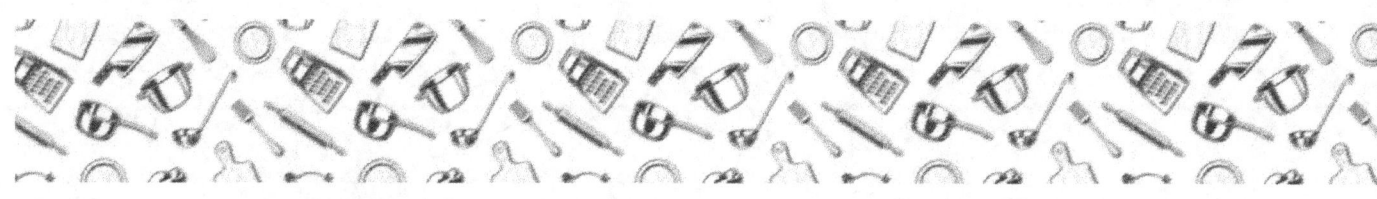

INGREDIENTS

a handful of fresh or frozen strawberries
1 banana
1.5 cup rolled oats
1.5 cup milk
a pinch of cinnamon 259

Nutritional Value: 234 calories per serving

DIRECTIONS

1. In a blender, Mix all the ingredients and blend until smooth.

Smoothies

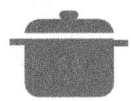 **Orange Coconut Smoothie**

COOKING: SERVES: 1

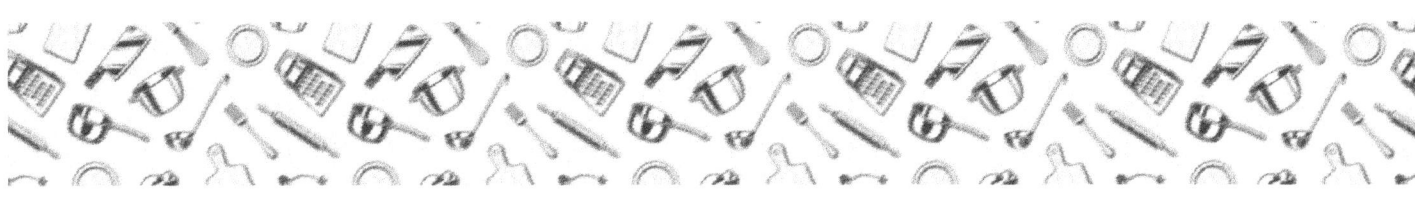

INGREDIENTS

2 1/2 cups hulled strawberries
1 orange, peeled
1/2 cup coconut milk
4 Ice cubes (optional)

Nutritional Value: 475 calories per serving

DIRECTIONS

1. Place all ingredients in a blender.

Smoothies

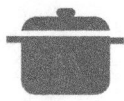 Peach Cinnamon Smoothie

COOKING: SERVES: 1

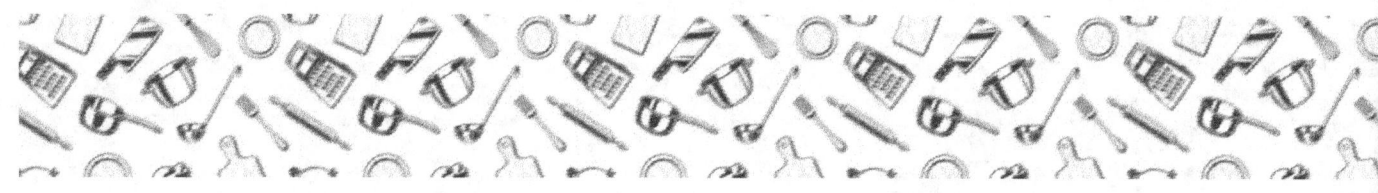

INGREDIENTS

2 ripe peaches
2 cups nonfat plain yogurt
3 tablespoons firmly packed brown sugar
1/4 teaspoon ground cinnamon
1 cup ice cubes

Nutritional Value: 123 calories per serving

DIRECTIONS

1. In a 2- to 3-quart pan over high heat, bring about 1-quart water to a boil. Immerse peaches in boiling water for 15 seconds; drain. When peaches are cool enough to touch, in 1 to 2 minutes, peel, pit, and cut into chunks. In a blender, combine peaches, yogurt, brown sugar, and cinnamon; whirl on high speed until smooth, about 1 minute. Add ice and whirl until smooth, about 2 minutes longer. Pour into tall glasses (at least 16-oz. size

Smoothies

Raspberry Peach Smoothie

COOKING: SERVES: 1

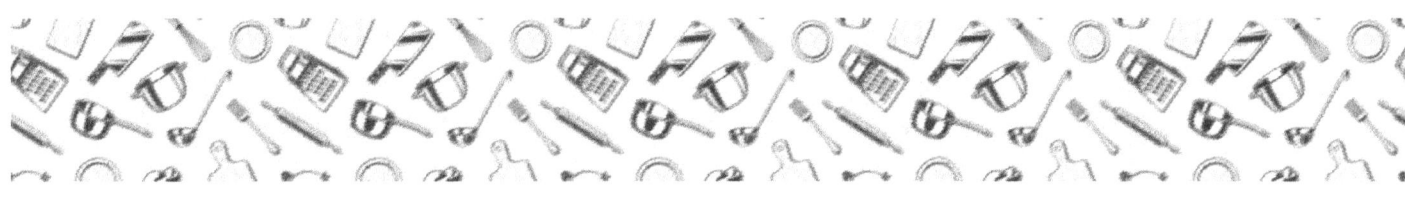

INGREDIENTS

10 oz frozen raspberries (in light syrup, thawed)
1 cup peach nectar
1/2 cup buttermilk
1 Tbsp. honey

Nutritional Value: 147 calories per serving

DIRECTIONS

1. Place all Ingredients in a blender and process until smooth. Serves 2.

Smoothies

 **Fruit Smoothie**

COOKING: SERVES: 1

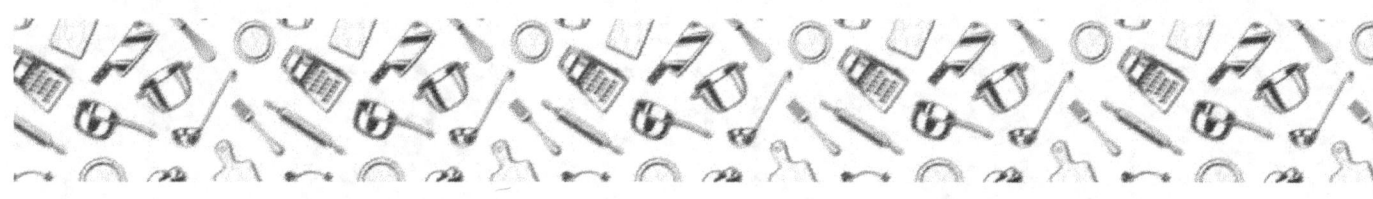

INGREDIENTS

1 frozen banana (best if cut into 1-inch -- chunks then frozen)
1/2 cup hulled strawberries (don't need to cut them up)
1/4 cup soy milk, orange juice or water cinnamon to taste

Nutritional Value: 210 calories per serving

DIRECTIONS

1. Add all of the Ingredients in a blender.

Smoothies

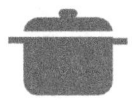

Apple Coconut Smoothie

COOKING: SERVES: 1

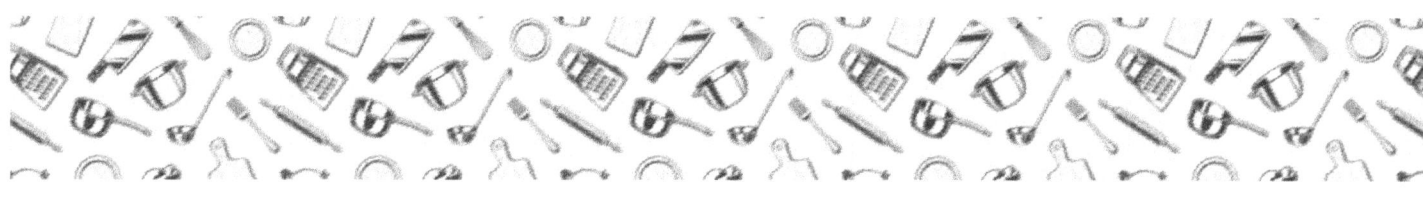

INGREDIENTS

4 c Apple juice
Coconut milk
1/2 Banana
1/4 teaspoon Ginger root -- fresh, peeled -grated
1/2 c -Crushed ice -- or 2 small ice - Cubes

Nutritional Value: 320 calories per serving

DIRECTIONS

1. Blend all until smooth.

Smoothies

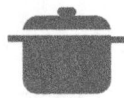 **High Fiber Smoothie**

COOKING: SERVES: 1

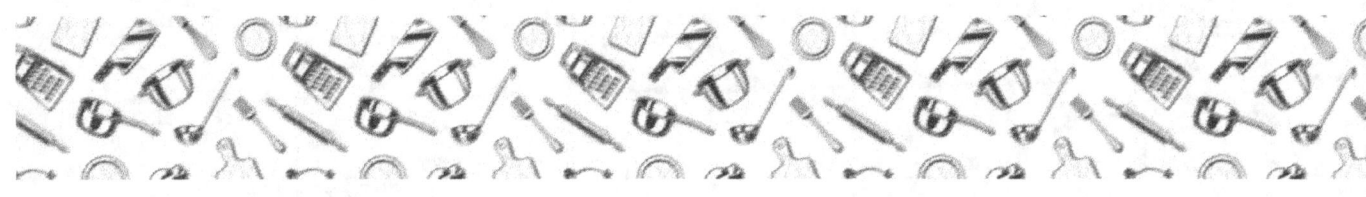

INGREDIENTS

1 cup blackberries
1 cup stemmed and halved strawberries
1 cup blueberries
1 cup low-fat vanilla soymilk
1/8 teaspoon ground cinnamon
3 ice cubes

Nutritional Value: 144 calories per serving

DIRECTIONS

1. Combine all ingredients in blender and whip until smooth. If berries are not fully ripe, add a little honey or sugar substitute for sweetness.

Smoothies

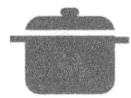

Apple Smoothie

COOKING: SERVES: 1

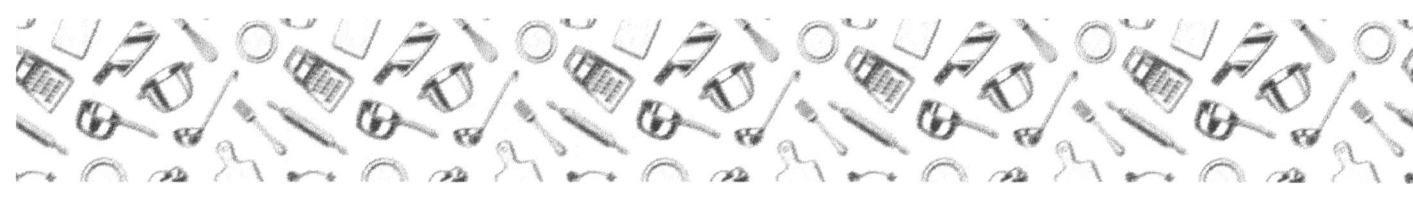

INGREDIENTS

2 cup Apple sauce
1 cup Apple cider
1 cup Orange juice
2 tablespoon maple syrup
1/2 teaspoon Nutmeg
1/2 teaspoon Cinnamon

Nutritional Value: 210 calories per serving

DIRECTIONS

1. Combine all ingredients in a blender and blend until smooth. Pour into glasses and serve.

Smoothies

 Triple Fruit Smoothie

COOKING: SERVES: 1

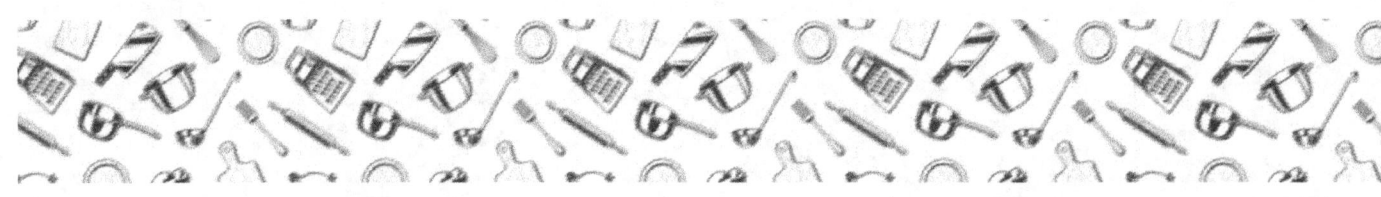

INGREDIENTS

1 banana
4 slices fresh or frozen peaches
4 fresh or frozen strawberries
10 ounces apple juice or cider
1/8 teaspoon cinnamon

Nutritional Value: 358 calories per serving

DIRECTIONS

1. Place all Ingredients in blender. Blend until smooth! Pour into chilled glass and garnish with fruit and a dash of cinnamon.

Smoothies

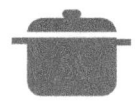

Strawberry Lemon Smoothie

COOKING:

SERVES: 1

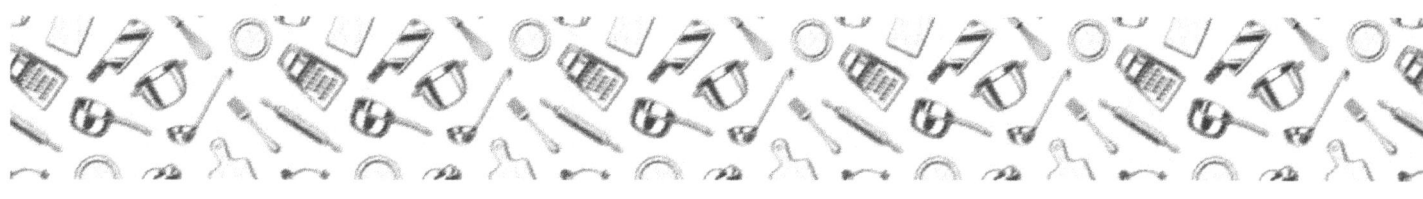

INGREDIENTS

2 cups lemonade
2 cups frozen strawberries
1 cup strawberry yogurt

Nutritional Value: 320 calories per serving

DIRECTIONS

1. Pour all liquid Ingredients into the blender. Add all frozen Ingredients. Blend at MIX setting for 30 seconds then blend at SMOOTH setting until smooth. While the machine is running, move the stir stick around counterclockwise to aid mixing. Serve immediately. Each recipe serves 3-5.

Smoothies

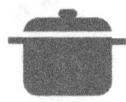

Morning Smoothie

COOKING:

SERVES: 1

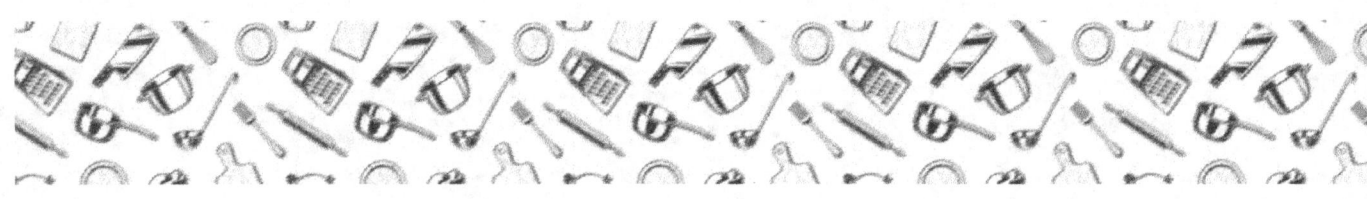

INGREDIENTS

2 Frozen Bananas
1 cup of sliced frozen peaches
1 cup of natural apple juice
½ cup of sliced strawberries

Nutritional Value: 300 calories per serving

DIRECTIONS

1. **Place all Ingredients in blender, mix and drink**

Smoothies

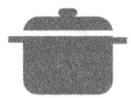

Pumpkin Smoothie

COOKING:

SERVES: 1

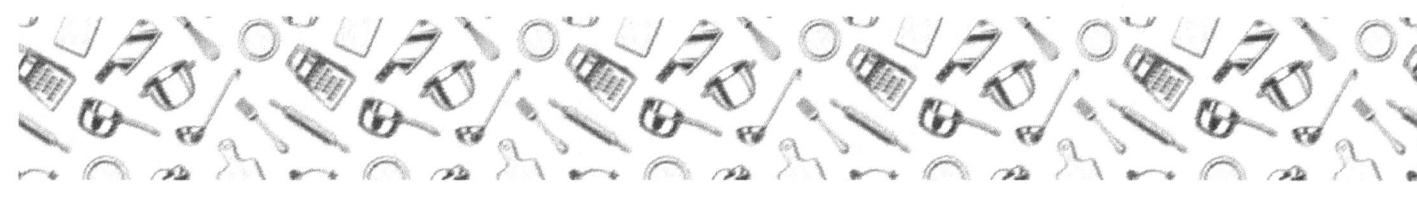

INGREDIENTS

1 3/4 cups pumpkin, canned -- chilled
12 ounces evaporated skim milk -- chilled
1 1/2 cups orange juice
1/2 cup banana -- sliced
1/3 cup brown sugar, packed

Nutritional Value: 217 calories per serving

DIRECTIONS

1. Place all ingredients in blender and blend well. If desired, serve over ice and sprinkle with cinnamon.

Smoothies

Paradise Smoothie

COOKING: SERVES: 1

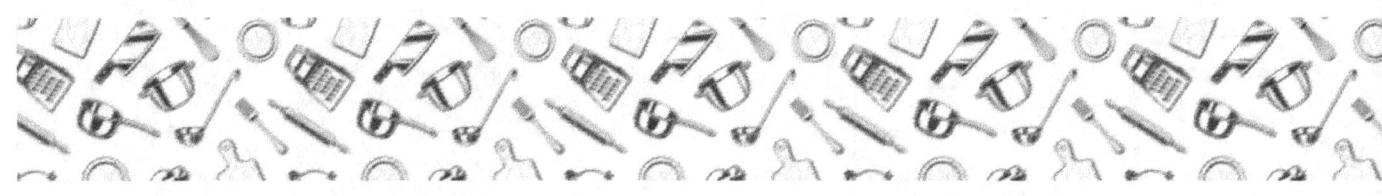

INGREDIENTS

1 1/2 cups pineapple-orange juice
1 cup sliced banana (about 1 medium)
1 cup ice cubes
3/4 cup diced pineapple
1/2 cup vanilla fat-free frozen yogurt
1 tablespoon flaked sweetened coconut

Nutritional Value: 244 calories per serving

DIRECTIONS

1. Combine all Ingredients in a blender, and process until smooth. Serve immediately.

Smoothies

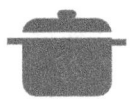

Honey Lime Fruit Cake

COOKING: SERVES: 1

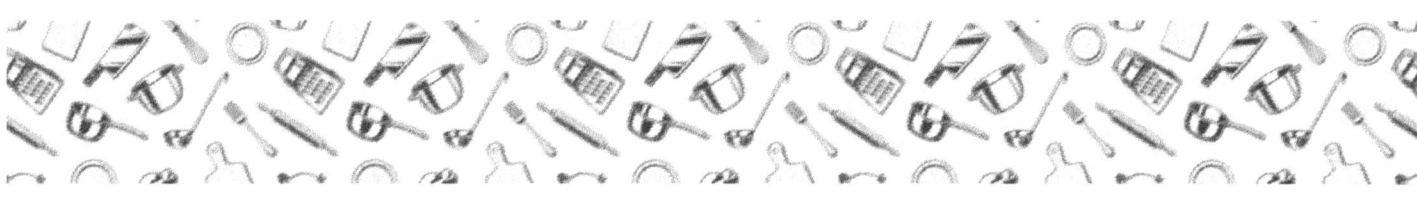

INGREDIENTS

2 bananas
1 cup blueberries
1 cup strawberries
Honey
1 cup lime
1 cup pine nuts

Nutritional Value: 115 calories per serving

DIRECTIONS

1. Hull and slice the strawberries and bananas.
2. Mix the blueberries, strawberries, and bananas in a bowl.
3. Cross over with the lime juice and honey.
4. Stir well and sprinkle with the nuts before serving.

Smoothies

Orange Smoothie

COOKING: SERVES: 1

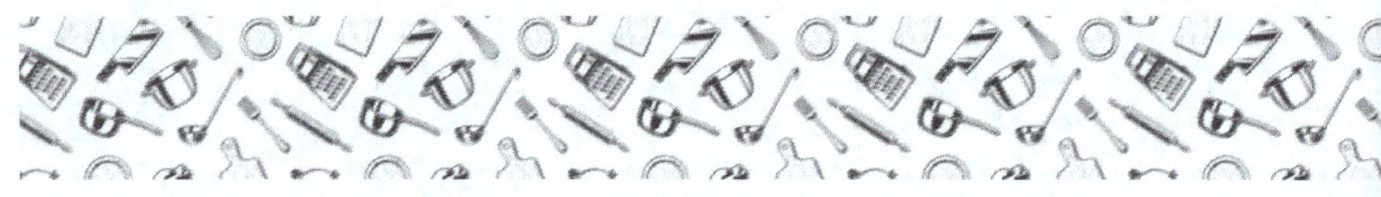

INGREDIENTS

1 medium banana, peeled and cut into 1-inch pieces
1 ripe peach, peeled, halved, pitted, and diced
1 cup raspberries
1 1/2 cups freshly squeezed orange juice
3 ice cubes

Nutritional Value:

123 calories per serving

DIRECTIONS

1. Combine all Ingredients in blender and whip until smooth.

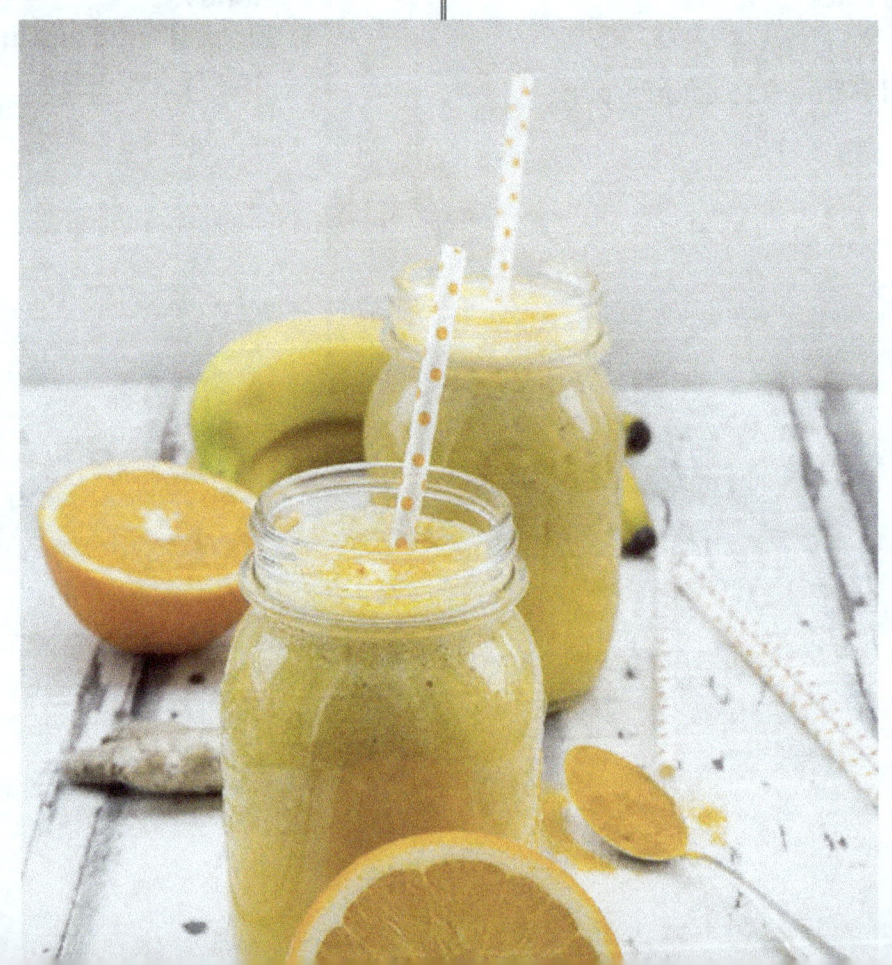

Smoothies

Banana Pineapple Smoothie

COOKING:

SERVES: 1

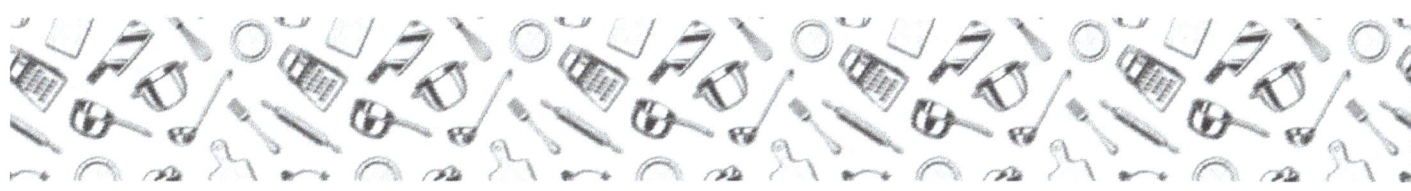

INGREDIENTS

1 banana
6 oz. light (reduced sugar) fat-free peach yogurt, frozen (This is one container of Yoplait)
6 oz. (1 can) Dole Pine-Orange-Banana juice

Nutritional Value: 147 calories per serving

DIRECTIONS

Put all Ingredients into blender. Blend until smoothie consistency is reached! If drink is too thick, add orange juice..

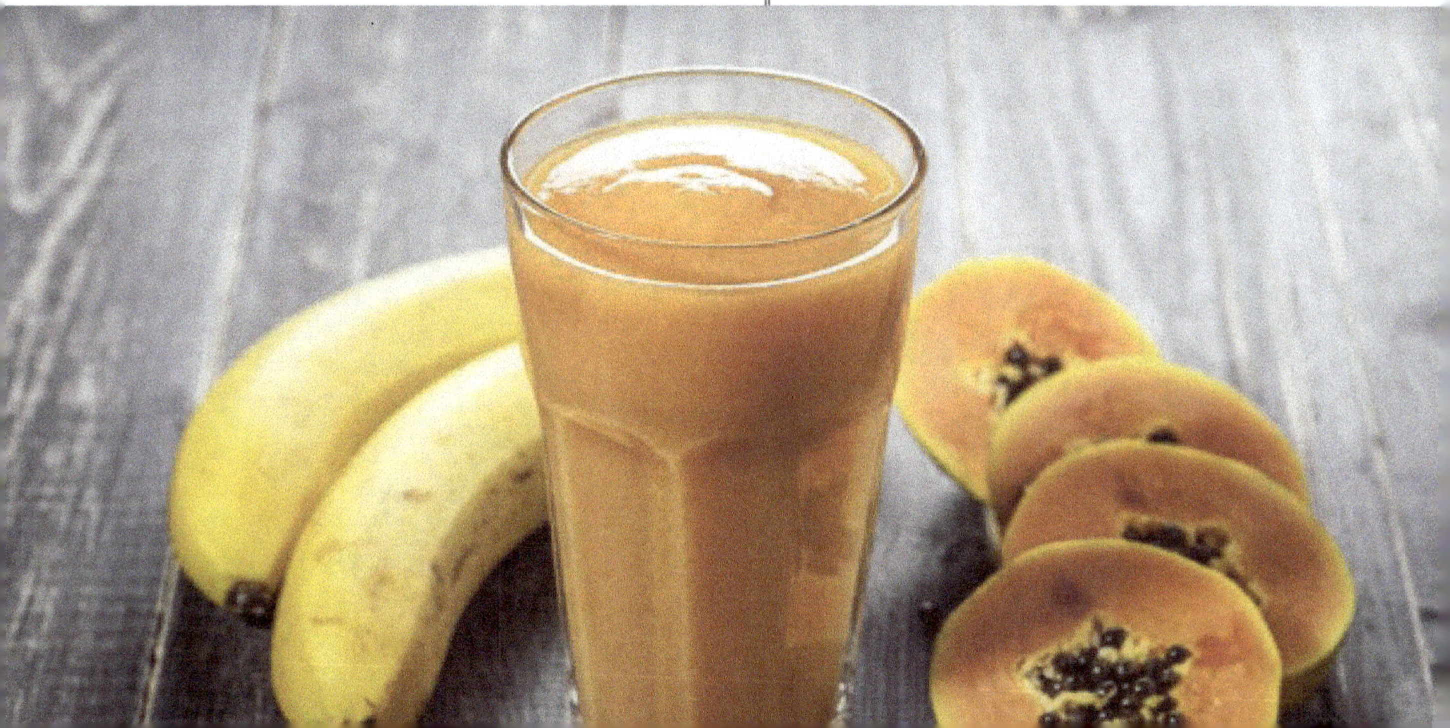

1.

Smoothies

Cappuccino Smoothie

COOKING: SERVES: 1

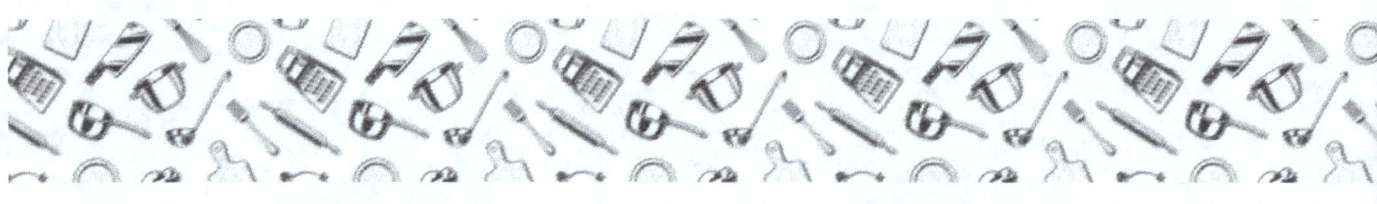

INGREDIENTS

3/4 cup chocolate milk, low-fat
1/3 cup fresh-brewed espresso
2 tablespoon chocolate syrup
1 1/2 cup nonfat coffee flavor frozen yogurt 1 cup raspberries
1/2 cup skim milk
1/4 teaspoon cocoa powder

Nutritional Value: 344 calories per serving

DIRECTIONS

1. Combine the chocolate milk, espresso, and chocolate syrup in a blender. Add the frozen yogurt and raspberries. Blend until smooth. Pour into glasses. Rinse out the blender container. Pour the milk into the blender and blend on high speed until frothy, about 15 seconds. Divide between the smoothies and sprinkle them with chocolate powder. Serves 2

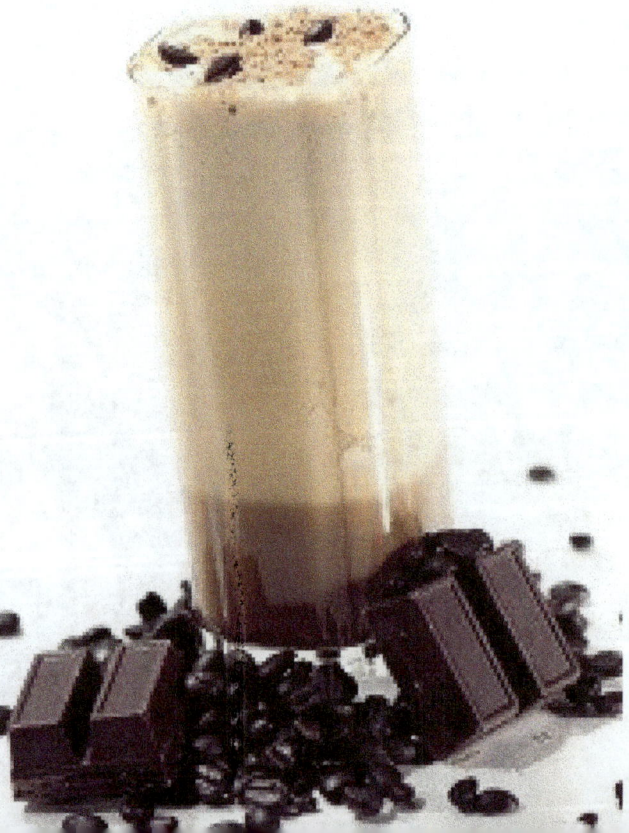

Smoothies

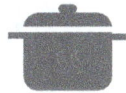

Peach Apple Smoothie

COOKING: SERVES: 1

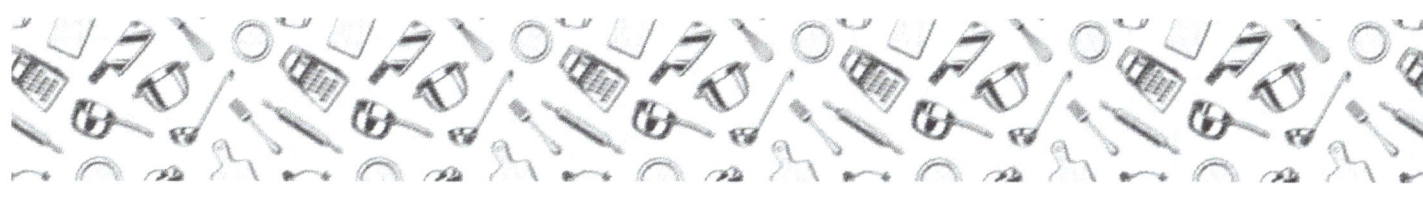

INGREDIENTS

1 fresh peach
1/3 cup non-fat milk
1/4 cup of frozen apple juice concentrate

Nutritional Value: 144 calories per serving

1.

DIRECTIONS

Peal 1 fresh peach. Cut it into thin slices. Put into a plastic bag with a zipper bag, lying flat. Put the plastic bag into the freezer for 1-2 hours. Take out 1/4 of the peaches and break them into pieces. Mix in a blender with 1/3 cup of milk and 1/4 cup of frozen apple juice concentrate. Cover and blend until smooth. pour into a glass and add more peach slices for peachy ice cubes!

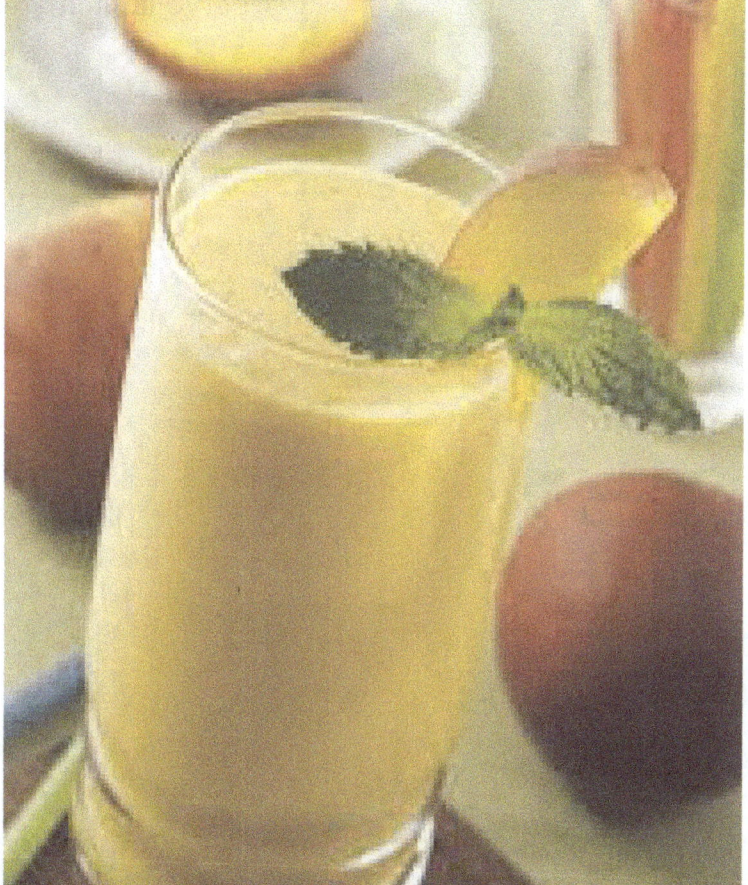

Smoothies

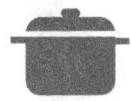

Mousse Mango

COOKING: 20 MIN

SERVES: 8

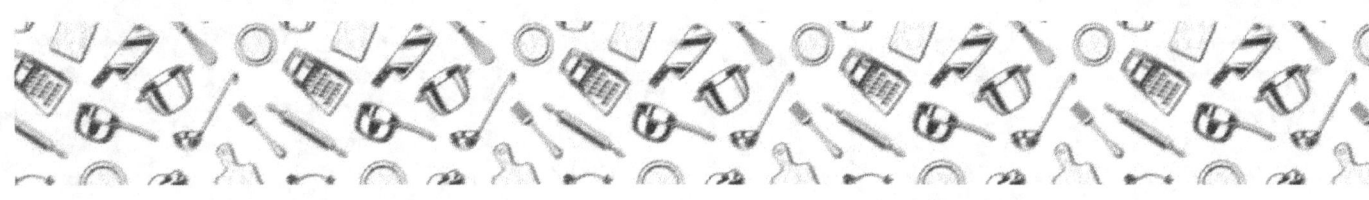

INGREDIENTS

3 ripe mangos
3 tablespoons agave syrup
1 cup coconut cream

Nutritional Value: 358 calories per serving

DIRECTIONS

1. Slice the mango to remove the stone.
2. Dice the flesh and place into a bowl. Mash them until smooth and puffy.
3. Add the coconut cream and whisk well. Whisk in the syrup. Spoon into the serving bowls.
4. Top off with a few chopped fruits and serve immediately.

www.ingramcontent.com/pod-product-compliance
Lightning Source LLC
Chambersburg PA
CBHW081354080526
44588CB00016B/2491